WHAT TO DO ABOUT THE FLU

Also by Pascal James Imperato

LAST ADVENTURE
Osa Johnson (editor)

BWANA DOCTOR

THE TREATMENT AND CONTROL OF INFECTIOUS
DISEASES IN MAN

THE CULTURAL HERITAGE OF AFRICA

A WIND IN AFRICA
A Story of Modern Medicine in Mali

HISTORICAL DICTIONARY OF MALI

WHAT TO DO
ABOUT THE FLU

Pascal James Imperato, M.D.

THOMAS CONGDON BOOKS

E. P. DUTTON & CO., INC. · NEW YORK

Library of Congress Cataloging in Publication Data

Imperato, Pascal James.
  What to do about the flu.

  "Thomas Congdon books."
  1. Influenza. 2. Influenza—Prevention.
I. Title. [DNLM: 1. Influenza—Prevention &
control—Popular works. WC515 134w]
RC150.I43   616.2'03   76-24919
ISBN: 0-525-23263-X

Published simultaneously in Canada
by Clarke, Irwin & Company Limited, Toronto and Vancouver

Acknowledgments

I wish to extend my sincerest thanks to Dr. John Stuart Marr, director of the Bureau of Preventable Diseases of the New York City Health Department, for his careful review of the manuscript and his helpful suggestions. My special thanks also go to David Obst, who first put forth the idea of this book and who helped it to happen. I wish to thank Mrs. Catherine Cowell, director of the Bureau of Nutrition, New York City Department of Health, for her help on the Anti-Flu Diet, and Mrs. Joyce Monteleone, Mrs. Sally Koch and Janet T. Lubow for preparing the typescript. And I wish to thank Dr. Lowell E. Bellin, Commissioner of Health, City of New York, for his support and encouragement.

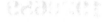

This Book is Dedicated with
All My Love to My Uncle
ALFRED A. IMPERATO, B.S., M.A., M.D.
Who Has Given Half a Century of Devoted
Service to Medicine and Mankind

Contents

to describe your symptoms over the telephone. What steps you can take to keep the flu from developing into pneumonia. The first signs of pneumonia. When you should consider going to the hospital for emergency treatment if you can't reach your doctor. What specific symptoms of pneumonia to look for in children.

Part II: MANKIND VERSUS THE FLU

The first recorded pandemic, in 1173 A.D. Influenza epidemics since then. The deadliest of all—the "Spanish Influenza." More recent epidemics—the Asian Flu of 1957, the Hong Kong Flu of 1968, and the London Flu of 1972.

There are three major types of influenza viruses—A, B and C. How these viruses, and their many subtypes, were discovered. How they change structure in order to survive when we are vaccinated or become immune through exposure. How new vaccines are developed and administered.

The new system for monitoring flu activity throughout the country. This system, which the author helped develop, is the only way to check on how much illness is being caused by flu virus. It coordinates reports from hospitals, large corporations, public service employers, and schools. Examples of this early warning system in operation, isolating viruses and developing vaccines before an epidemic can mushroom.

Why Swine flu is distinct from the flu viruses now known. Its peculiar characteristics. The outbreaks that have already occurred. Why this strain is potentially fatal. How much illness and death it can be expected to cause. How President Ford's decision was reached. How the medical community has reacted. What kinds of activities can be expected in cities across the country.

Part III: APPENDICES

What role diet plays in flu prevention and treatment. A diet that will equip you to fight off the flu and other respiratory infections.

The ten essential steps to take to escape the flu.

How to treat yourself right if your preventive measures have been in vain. The ten basics of flu treatment.

Why This Book

You may be one of those people who think you can't do much to prevent the flu. You tell yourself that you'll either catch it or you won't, so you leave it to fate.

You'll be happy to hear that you're wrong. There are plenty of things you can do to arm yourself against the flu—to make it less likely you'll get it. What's more, there are simple, practical ways to ease your suffering if you do get sick. You don't have to just lie there and moan.

The aim of this book is to change you from a passive, fatalistic flu victim and flu spreader to an active flu preventer and flu therapist. Instead of bringing the flu home to your family, you can help keep them from getting it. You don't have to infect your friends or office associates. And you don't have to wonder with a fevered brain about the right thing to do to treat your sickness.

This book should help you against any flu, in any year. (Even if you are vaccinated against a serious virus such as the Swine flu, you can get it anyway, and there may be other flus around that same season.) There will always be a flu bug. They are hardy and resourceful viruses that have survived so long—at least a thousand years—because they know how to get to you and me. As we build up immunity to specific viruses, they shift and change their structure, enabling their descendants to pass through our wall of immunity and start new epidemics. The flu is persistent—but it is not invincible. You can fight back.

Much of the advice offered in this book is based on my years of experience in answering questions from my patients, from private physicians (I am a public health doctor specializing in preventing epidemics), and from the general public. I have tried to cover the major issues involving the flu, but there are of course variations in the way the flu behaves, from person to person and from year to year. If you do catch it, don't wait. Call your doctor.

PASCAL JAMES IMPERATO, M.D.

Part One

YOUR FIGHT
AGAINST THE FLU

CHAPTER I

Avoiding the Flu

Did you have the flu last year? If you did, then you know what a hassle it involves—body aches and pains, sore throat, runny nose, weakness and dizziness. You swallowed at least a bottle of aspirin and maybe some expensive antibiotics. You drank gallons of soups and juices. You used countless handkerchiefs and tissues. You tossed and turned, night after night. All because of the flu. You missed work, maybe for as long as a couple of weeks, and you worried about your job while, in the meantime, your family and friends worried about *you*. If you have children, you probably gave it to them, and they were absent from school for much longer than you'd have liked. What a painful, costly, time-consuming phenomenon this disease is!

From every aspect, then, it's better to prevent the flu than to treat it. The first step is to learn some basic facts about flu prevention, including some dos and don'ts.

Q. What is the flu?
A. The flu is a contagious disease caused by a group of viruses.
Q. How many types of flu viruses are there?
A. There are three broad types of flu virus, called A, B and C. Types A and B have been the cause of most illness over the years. Epidemics due to Type A are more frequent and more serious than those due to Type B.

Q. What are the symptoms of the flu?

A. Flu symptoms vary greatly from person to person. The average person who gets the flu usually experiences fever, chills, cough, body aches and pains, and weakness. Sore throat and running nose tend to occur a day or two after the illness starts. Some people who get infected with the flu virus do not become ill at all. This is called an *inapparent infection.* For a variety of reasons they are resistant to the flu virus.

Q. Is the flu known by other names?

A. Yes. The flu is commonly called the grippe or influenza, which is its scientific name.

Q. How long does a bout of the flu last?

A. Most people recover from the acute symptoms within two to seven days. Often people feel weak and tire easily for another ten days or so after recovering.

Q. What are the complications of the flu?

A. The major complication of the flu is pneumonia which fortunately occurs in only a small percentage of flu patients. Bronchitis and infections of the sinuses and the middle ear are less serious complications.

Q. Can you get the flu more than once in the same year?

A. Yes. It is unusual for this to happen, however. If someone becomes ill with the A flu virus in January, he could still become ill with the B flu virus in the spring. The viruses are different and having one flu does not always build up your immunity to the others. The viruses also change periodically, so that the A virus you had in January may be replaced by a new A virus in November. Infection from the first may not protect against the second. You will not have the *same* flu twice in the same year, however.

Q. Can you confuse the flu with other diseases?

A. Yes. A number of other viral diseases produce symptoms similar to those of the flu. You may have such an infection, recover from it and then catch the flu. This might make you think you had the flu twice when you really only had it once.

Q. How does a bout of the flu protect you from subsequent attacks?

A. The flu virus makes your body produce protective substances called *antibodies*. These substances circulate in the blood and are found in the cells of the body. From then on, whenever the flu virus enters the body, they destroy it.

Q. How serious a disease is the flu?

A. The flu is a moderately severe disease from which most people completely recover within three to seven days. It is a very serious disease among persons over the age of sixty-five and persons of any age who have one or more chronic diseases. These chronic conditions are (1) heart disease, such as rheumatic or congenital heart disease, (2) chronic lung disease like asthma, chronic bronchitis, emphysema and tuberculosis, (3) diabetes mellitus and (4) chronic kidney disease. People in these categories are called "high risk" because they are more likely to develop potentially fatal complications. They should receive a flu shot every year if there are no contraindications.

Q. Do people die from the flu?

A. Yes, but most deaths are due to complications, not to the flu itself. Considering the large number of people who are ill with the flu each year, only a small proportion die as a result of the disease or its complications.

Q. How is the flu spread?

A. The influenza virus that causes the flu is present in the fluids of the nose, mouth and throat of a person who is coming down with the disease. These fluids are sprayed out into the surrounding air in fine droplets when the person talks, coughs or sneezes. They can then be breathed into the noses and mouths of healthy people nearby. The virus is also present in the handkerchiefs and paper tissues used by flu patients. Healthy people who touch these items and then touch their mouths or noses can catch the infection. The flu spreads easily in crowded places like buses, elevators and barracks.

Q. How long does it take to develop symptoms once you have been exposed to the flu?

A. Once you are infected, symptoms develop quickly—within one to three days. You may, of course, be exposed to someone with the flu and not catch it. Or you may catch it and not develop any symptoms.

Q. How long is the flu contagious?

A. If you have the flu, you can potentially spread it to others during the first three days or so after your own symptoms appear. Some flu victims continue to shed the virus from their noses and throats for several days after that.

Q. Do certain people catch the flu or does everyone?

A. Everyone is susceptible to catching any given flu except those who have already had it that year and most of those who have received flu shots.

Q. During what months of the year is the flu most common?

A. Outbreaks and epidemics of the flu due to Type A tend to occur in the Temperate Zone (which includes the United States) between the months of November and February. Type B infections often occur in the Temperate Zone during the spring. In the tropics Type A and Type B outbreaks and epidemics occur at any time of the year.

Q. How often do epidemics of the flu occur?

A. Epidemics due to Type A influenza virus tend to occur every two to three years and those due to Type B virus every four to six years.

Q. Why do flu epidemics occur at these intervals?

A. New virus strains of both Type A and Type B tend to develop every few years. Sometimes these new strains are very different from those which previously infected the population. These new strains can cause large epidemics because people have never been exposed to them and consequently have no immunity against them.

Q. Why do so many flu epidemics occur during the winter months?

A. All the reasons for this are not yet known. During the winter months in the Temperate Zone, the natural defense mechanisms of the nose, throat and respiratory tract are weakened by the cold weather. This makes it easier for flu viruses to invade the body. Also, people are indoors more during the winter, in crowded conditions that make transmission of the flu a simple matter. Another factor is central heating—in overheated apartments and houses, the relative humidity tends to be low. The dry air weakens the natural defenses of the nose, throat and respiratory tract. A similar phenomenon can be seen in some parts of Africa near the southern edge of the Sahara. Flu outbreaks often occur there between the months of February and June, which is the hot dry season. There too the dry air breaks down the defenses of the respiratory tract and, in addition, the virus is helped to spread by the dust of the region.

Q. Does one strain of flu virus cause more serious illness than others?

A. Yes, Type A virus infections (Swine flu, for example) tend to cause more serious illness than those due to Type B virus. But in general, the seriousness of a bout of the flu often has more to do with the individual's response to the infection than with the virus itself. Someone who is seriously run down, or has a chronic disease, will suffer more than an average, healthy person.

Flu Vaccine

Q. Who should receive flu shots?

A. Annual vaccination against the flu is recommended for people of all ages who have any of the following chronic disabling medical conditions: (1) diabetes mellitus or any other metabolic disease, (2) chronic lung disease such as asthma, chronic bronchitis, cystic fibrosis, emphysema or advanced tuberculosis, (3) congenital or rheumatic heart disease, or heart disease due to high blood pressure or hardening of the arteries.

In addition, it is advisable to immunize people over the age of sixty-five, especially if they have chronic diseases of the lungs and heart. Routine annual vaccination of the entire population is not recommended, except when a new and especially virulent strain appears, like Swine flu.

Q. Who should *not* get a flu shot?

A. Flu vaccines are made from viruses grown on eggs, so anyone who is allergic to eggs should not ordinarily be vaccinated. Nor should flu vaccinations be given to anyone who is ill with an acute infection of any kind, such as measles or a sore throat.

Q. If I receive a flu shot, can I still get the flu?

A. Yes, it is possible that you could get the flu anyway. The vaccine protects from 70 to 90 percent of those who receive it, but only against the strain of the virus from which the vaccine is made. Some protection is given against related strains, but usually not against new strains. So if a new strain comes on the scene, the vaccine made from the previous year's strain may not give much protection.

Q. When a new strain appears, why can't a vaccine be made against it immediately?

A. It takes about six months to produce sufficient quantities of a new flu vaccine. When a new strain is identified as being the cause of a large epidemic, vaccine production is started at once, but it's already too late for the first year's victims. By the time the vaccine is ready, six months later, the epidemic will have run its course. An exception has been the Swine flu virus, which was isolated and identified before it had caused a widespread epidemic. Vaccine production has already begun, and will be ready in time if an epidemic occurs.

Q. What is the duration of protection given by a flu shot?

A. This varies from one person to another and with the vaccine. On the average, a flu shot protects for about six months.

Q. Can you get the flu from a flu shot?

A. No. Flu vaccines are made from killed viruses. In order to develop the flu, live flu viruses must be present.

Q. What time of year is best for getting a flu shot?

A. For maximum protection in the Temperate Zone, get your flu shot by October. This way, when the flu season begins in November, you will be protected.

Q. Should pregnant women receive flu shots?

A. In an ordinary year, pregnant women are not normally given flu immunizations unless their doctors think they should be. Pregnant women can receive flu shots if their obstetricians or family physicians think they are indicated.

Q. Should children receive flu shots?

A. Unless persons under the age of sixty-five are suffering from the chronic medical conditions I have described above, they are not usually given flu shots. In the Swine flu immunization programs now being established, there are no plans for immunizing very young children.

Q. Who should be immunized against the Swine flu?

A. In the opinion of many experts, everyone should be immunized against the Swine flu, except children under the age of six, or people who are allergic to eggs or who should avoid the vaccine for medical reasons that their family doctors would know about.

Q. Can you develop adverse reactions after a flu shot?

A. Yes. In a recent study it was found that a small percentage of those receiving flu shots suffered generalized side reactions during the first twenty–four hours. Four percent had chills, 4 percent fever, 6 percent aches and pains and 12 percent headache. These reactions are similar to symptoms of the flu itself, which may contribute to the popular misconception that a flu shot gives you a mild case of the flu. This is not true. Most of these side reactions disappeared by the second day, unlike flu symptoms, which continue much longer. And more common than these reactions in the study were local reactions at the site of the inoculation, 40 percent having some pain, 47 percent tenderness and 9 percent swelling within the first day. Most of these problems cleared up by the third day. Rarely, someone who is allergic to eggs or some other component of the vaccine can develop an acute and serious allergic reaction, which can be fatal if not treated promptly. This type of reaction is called an *anaphylactic reaction.*

Q. How many flu shots are needed in a year?

A. Generally, only one shot a year is necessary since most vaccines contain both Types A and B killed virus. If the vaccine contains only Type A, then you will need to get a second shot with Type B vaccine. In 1974 many people received two shots: the first vaccine contained Types A and B, and the second contained the B/Hong Kong strain which had just appeared. The Hong Kong vaccine had been developed and produced in time to be effective against Influenza B, but not in time to be combined in one shot with the then-existing vaccines.

Q. What is meant by monovalent and bivalent flu vaccines?

A. A monovalent flu vaccine is one which contains only one type of killed virus, either Type A or Type B. A bivalent vaccine is one which contains two types of killed virus, usually Type A and Type B. The bivalent flu vaccines are the kind more widely used today.

Q. What kind of vaccine is being used against Swine flu?

A. Two types of vaccine are being used against Swine flu. The first is a bivalent vaccine which contains killed viruses of Swine flu and the Victoria strain of Type A influenza, the one that has been widespread in 1975 and 1976. This bivalent vaccine is being given to all those who usually qualify by reason of age or ill health to receive annual flu immunizations. The second type is a monovalent vaccine containing only the killed Swine flu virus, and it is being offered to the remainder of the population.

What You Should Do and Not Do to Prevent the Flu

Q. Does avoiding exposure to bad weather prevent the flu?

A. Yes, in a non-specific way. Exposure to wet and cold weather tends to lower your body's resistance and make you more susceptible to infection.

Q. Does avoiding excessive exposure outdoors on windy days prevent the flu?

A. Yes. The flu virus can be carried in wind currents. Also, winds tend to damage the lining of the nose and throat, making you more susceptible.

Q. Will wearing a face mask help?

A. No. Face masks are not effective in filtering out the small flu virus. The virus can easily pass through them. During the great flu epidemic of 1918 face masks became mandatory in many parts of the world. But they did not stop the spread of the flu.

Q. Will frequent hand-washing help prevent the flu?

A. Routine hand-washing is a good hygienic habit and is effective in preventing the flu. It is amazing how often we put our hands to our faces during the day. Hand-washing removes germs of all kinds and reduces the risk of our infecting ourselves.

Q. Friends have just invited me to their home for dinner. They have both just recovered from the flu. Should I go?

A. No. You should politely decline the invitation. Some people stop shedding the flu virus within a few days of getting sick, but others are contagious several days longer. Postpone your dinner for another week, to be on the safe side.

Q. I have been invited to a friend's home for cocktails. One of their children has the flu but no one else has had it. Would it be safe for me to go?

A. It would be better not to go, even if you were to avoid contact with their sick child. Chances are good that other members of the family are in the early stages of the flu and could pass it on to you.

Q. My fiancée is sick with the flu. Should I visit her?

A. No. If you have been seeing her regularly and were with her the first day of her illness, you have already been exposed to the virus. But you may not get the flu as a result, depending on whether you are already immune and whether you breathed in the virus. Further exposure will only increase your chances of contracting it.

If you have not seen her since the day before she became ill, you have not been exposed to the virus. Why deliberately take chances now? Instead of visiting, give her a call by phone. If she really loves you she will not want you to get the flu.

Q. Is it safe to kiss someone who has the flu?

A. No. Kissing is one of the most efficient ways by which the flu is spread.

Q. How safe is it to shake hands with someone who has the flu?

A. It is not very safe at all. His hand may be contaminated with flu virus. Even more important, shaking hands would bring you into close physical contact and expose you to the flu virus that would fill the air as the other person talked, coughed and sneezed.

Q. When a flu epidemic starts, can I avoid catching it by moving to an isolated part of the country?

A. No. Moving to a less populated area would *lessen* the risk of your catching the flu. But eventually the flu virus spreads everywhere. During the great 1918 epidemic the flu even reached Eskimos living in isolated parts of Alaska. It is almost a certainty that the flu would eventually find you in your rural hideaway.

Q. Does avoiding crowds protect you from the flu?

A. Yes. In fact, you should make every effort to avoid crowds during a flu epidemic. It is well known that the flu virus spreads more easily in crowded places.

Q. If someone next to me on a bus is sneezing, should I move away?

A. Yes. If he is coming down with the flu, your chances of catching it are increased if you remain near him. By moving to another part of the bus, you reduce the risk of picking up his infection. He may have nothing more than a head cold or an allergy, but you have everything to gain and nothing to lose by moving far away from him.

Q. If someone on an elevator is coughing a great deal, will I prevent the flu by holding my breath or by getting off at the next floor?

A. If that person has the flu, you will reduce your chances of contracting it by getting off at the next floor. Holding your breath might be helpful for a few seconds, but prolonged breath holding is neither a safe nor an efficient method of protecting yourself from the virus.

Q. Should flu patients cover their coughs and sneezes with a handkerchief?

A. Yes. By so doing they substantially reduce the spread of the flu virus.

Q. How useful are antiseptic mouthwashes in preventing the flu?

A. Although mouthwashes are good for oral hygiene, they do not deter the flu virus.

Q. Are there any antibiotics that can be taken to prevent the flu?

A. No. Antibiotics have no direct effect on flu viruses.

Q. Are there any drugs that can be used to prevent the flu?

A. There are some drugs that effectively kill flu viruses. But these often cause serious side reactions like nausea, vomiting and headache that can be worse than the flu itself. Therefore I do not recommend their use.

Q. Is it safe to sleep in the bedroom of a person who has just recovered from the flu?

A. Yes, provided the room has been aired and cleaned and the bed linens replaced.

Q. When a family member has the flu, should his dishes and eating utensils be segregated?

A. If his dishes and eating utensils are washed in hot water, they need not be segregated. In homes where this is not possible, they should be kept separate.

Q. Should a person who is sick with the flu mail letters to friends?

A. Unless it is absolutely necessary, it would be better if he didn't. If he must, the letters should be aired for a few hours before they are mailed. This assures that any flu virus on the paper is dead, as the virus does not survive long on such material.

Q. A friend of mine is ill with the flu. If I visit him, do I risk bringing it home to my wife and children?

A. Yes. You could contract it yourself and then spread it to your family.

Q. Can you get the flu from drinking at public water fountains?

A. This is unlikely. Someone with the flu would have to have contaminated the spout by breathing on it or touching it with his mouth. Then you would have to touch the spout with your lips soon afterwards.

Q. Can you get the flu by eating peanuts from a common bowl at a bar?

A. Probably not. Peanuts are not a favorable site for the survival of the flu virus.

Q. Does a common drinking cup in a bathroom help to spread the flu?

A. Yes. Such cups should not be used.

Q. Does sucking on medicated lozenges prevent the flu?

A. No, it doesn't.

Q. A week ago I was exposed to someone with the flu. Can I still come down with it?

A. It takes from one to three days to develop symptoms of the flu after exposure. So you will not come down with the flu at this late date from that exposure. You can still get the flu, however, if you are exposed to someone else with the disease.

Q. Can you get the flu from the drinking glasses and eating utensils in restaurants?

A. Only if they are improperly washed, which is not unusual in some establishments.

Q. Can you get the flu from eating food sold by street vendors?

A. If a vendor's level of personal hygiene is poor and if his foods are openly displayed and thus easily contaminated, you can be running a real risk of contracting not only the flu but possibly other infections as well.

Q. Do calesthenics help to prevent the flu?

A. No, not directly. But they do keep you physically fit and enhance your body's resistance to infection.

Q. Does smoking prevent the flu?

A. No. In fact, smoking injures the respiratory tract and makes you more susceptible to the flu and its complications.

Q. Can you get the flu from using public toilets?

A. No.

Q. Can you get the flu from handling the clothing and bed linens of someone who has it?

A. Yes, if they have been recently contaminated with fluids from the person's mouth and nose.

Q. Does spitting in public spread the flu?

A. Yes, if the person spitting has the flu and is spitting out the virus.

Q. Does wearing a scarf and sweater prevent the flu?

A. No, not directly, but wearing these items protects the body from cold weather and helps you resist flu infection.

Q. My husband just came down with the flu. If I get a flu shot right away, will it prevent me from getting the flu?

A. Unfortunately, a flu shot will not help you. It requires about two weeks for the body to respond to a flu shot with good levels of antibodies. Since the disease takes three days at most to develop, it is likely that you have already been infected. If you have *not* been infected, you can take some precautions. Don't come too close to your husband while caring for him. Cheer him up without kissing him. Sleep in another bedroom, or on the living room couch—anywhere but in the same room with your 'patient.

Q. Someone coughed in my face on the bus. Will I get the flu?

A. You might, if he had the flu and if you are susceptible to the infection. Otherwise you will not. If three days pass and you develop no symptoms, you can assume you did not contract the flu.

Q. Should a person sick with the flu use the family telephone?

A. It would be preferable if he didn't, since he could contaminate the receiver.

Q. Can you get the flu from the receivers of public telephones?

A. It's possible, if you use a phone immediately after someone who is sick with the flu.

Q. During a flu epidemic should I go to the movies?

A. It would be best not to, since the disease spreads easily in crowded places like movie theaters.

Q. Do flies and mosquitoes spread the flu?

A. There is no evidence that mosquitoes transmit the flu viruses. A fly may mechanically pick up the flu virus on its legs by walking on a contaminated handkerchief. It might then spread the virus by walking on the rim of a drinking glass or by landing on someone's legs. However, while all this is theoretically possible, such modes of transmission have not been conclusively verified.

Q. Can I get the flu from washing my clothes and bed linens in a public laundromat?

A. No, the temperature of the water used in the machines will kill any flu virus present in the machine or on the materials being washed.

Q. Can I spread the flu among my family by washing our clothes and sheets together in our basement washing machine?

A. No, the hot water used in the machine will kill any flu virus that the sick member of the family had shed on clothes or bed linen.

Children and the Flu

Q. Is the flu a serious disease in children?

A. Generally, the flu is a relatively mild to moderate disease in children.

Q. Should I have my young son immunized against the flu every year?

A. No, not unless he has one of the chronic medical problems discussed earlier.

Q. My daughter recovered from the flu yesterday and feels okay. She would like to go to the movies with some of her friends. Should I let her go?

A. No, you should not, because she could possibly spread the disease to her friends and others in the theater. It is best to wait at least three days after recovery before going into crowded places.

Q. My son is a star of the high school football and wrestling teams. There is a flu epidemic in town. Should I make him curtail his sports activities?

A. No, it is not necessary to do so if he is getting adequate rest and has a nutritious diet.

Q. My son just recovered from the flu and wants to resume his swimming lessons. Should I allow him to do so?

A. No, because he could spread the infection to others and jeopardize his own health by exerting himself before he is fully recovered. It is best to wait about two weeks after recovery before engaging in swimming.

Q. My son is on the high school football team. He just recovered from the flu and his coach wants him to resume playing. Should I allow this?

A. No, you should not, because your son may still be shedding the flu virus and could spread it to his teammates. Also, he may not be fully recovered. It is best to wait about one to two weeks after the last day of fever before resuming vigorous sports activities. This allows time for more complete recuperation.

Q. Does closing schools during flu epidemics prevent the spread of the disease?

A. No, this is not a useful measure. For one thing, kids who are kept home from school will probably go out in the street and mix with other kids anyway, so they won't be isolated from the possibility of infection. Besides, children who contract the flu usually get off lightly. During the great 1918 Spanish influenza epidemic, the morbidity rate among children was extremely low compared to the number of adults who died from the disease. When you weigh the negative results of keeping a child out of school against the risk he runs if he goes to school, it's better to let him attend.

Q. Can children get the flu from eating unwrapped candy?

A. Probably not (although it would be best if they didn't buy such candies, since a number of other infections can be passed on that way; watch out on Halloween).

Q. It is a very rainy day. My son's high school football coach wants the team to practice in the rain on a muddy field to harden them up. Should I let my son do this?

A. The coach's intentions may be sincere but his methods are unwise. Unnecessary exposure of children to rain, wet mud and cold temperatures will reduce their physical resistance and make them more susceptible to the flu and other infections. It would be best not to let your son participate and to try to get the coach to call the practice off.

Q. One of my children has the flu. Should I keep the others home from school?

A. No. There is no medical reason to do so. But try to keep your other children out of the sick room, and make sure the sick child eats his meals in his room, not at the table with the family.

Q. How long should my seven-year-old son be kept home out of school after he has recovered from the flu?

A. It is best to keep him home for at least five days after his temperature has returned to normal. By that time most children are fully recovered, feel physically fit and are not shedding the flu virus. If your child has had a particularly severe case of the flu then it would be best to be guided by the advice of your family physician. It may be necessary to keep him home longer.

Q. When children perspire a great deal from vigorous physical exercise, are they more susceptible to the flu?

A. Not necessarily, unless they then get chilled in the cold weather and experience a sudden reduction of body temperature. Such an abrupt change in body temperature tends to lower resistance to infection.

Q. Can children get the flu from sitting on brick or concrete steps?

A. No, but if they do so in the winter, they can get chilled and lower their physical resistance to the flu virus.

Q. A classmate of my son baked cookies at home and gave them out to the class yesterday. Today we learned she is home with the flu. What should I do?

A. It is unlikely that the other children became infected from eating the cookies. It is more likely that the girl has passed the flu on to her classmates directly. There are no measures you can take, except to observe your own child during the next three days. If no symptoms develop, then he did not become infected from either the cookies or his sick classmate. He could, of course, contract the flu later on from someone else.

Q. My thirteen-year-old daughter came home from school and said that some of her classmates have the "intestinal flu." What is this disease?

A. "Intestinal flu" is a term widely used by people to describe a number of different infections which cause gastrointestinal symptoms like nausea, vomiting and diarrhea. It is not influenza, which primarily affects the respiratory tract. "Intestinal flu" is not a scientifically acceptable term and should not be used.

Q. There is a flu epidemic going on. My son's high school football team is in the habit of drinking salt solution out of a common canteen. The coach told me that they don't touch their lips to the canteen when they drink. What should I do?

A. This is a common practice, but an unwise one. The coach may think they don't touch their lips to the canteen, but they probably do quite often. Even if they don't, any of the boys who are coming down with the flu are sure to contaminate the canteen simply by breathing on the opening. The coach should make each player bring his own canteen.

Dietary Habits and the Flu

Q. Does taking Vitamin C help to prevent the flu?

A. Many experts think that Vitamin C does cut down on the frequency of colds and other virus infections of the respiratory tract. Although there is as yet no *conclusive* scientific evidence which convinces the entire medical world that Vitamin C prevents the flu, there is abundant empirical evidence that it does. It would certainly be a reasonable preventive measure to employ.

Q. What kinds of foods will give me added protection against the flu?

A. A well-balanced diet consisting of protein, carbohydrate and fat results in a good state of nutrition. This in turn serves as a good defense against the flu. (See The Anti-Flu Diet, at the end of this book.)

Q. Should I take vitamin supplements to prevent the flu?

A. If you are eating a well-balanced diet it is unlikely that you need to take vitamin pills in addition. But some medical experts do advocate taking Vitamin C, as I have already indicated.

Q. Do alcoholic beverages prevent the flu?

A. Many would like to believe that alcoholic beverages are a good defense against the flu, but they are not. Since the flu viruses enter the respiratory tract and alcohol the gastrointestinal tract, the twain never meet.

Q. Do laxatives prevent the flu?

A. No, they do not.

1920689

Q. Will drinking hot beverages like coffee and tea protect me from the flu?

A. No, it will not.

Q. Does drinking iced beverages when you are perspiring and overheated dispose you to the flu?

A. There is no evidence that it does. But in general, abrupt changes of body temperature tend to weaken physical defenses. So one should drink such beverages slowly when the body is overheated.

Q. Is crash dieting during a flu epidemic wise?

A. Crash dieting is viewed by most medical experts as unwise in general. If you do it during a flu epidemic, you will deprive yourself of vitamins and nutrients that your body must have to defend itself against infection.

Q. Does a vegetarian diet make you prone to the flu?

A. No, it does not, provided that it is balanced with the required proportions of protein, carbohydrate, fat, vitamins and minerals.

Q. I have heard from many Europeans that mineral water taken daily is a good way to prevent the flu. Is this true?

A. No. Bottled mineral water is widely used in many parts of the world for the treatment and prevention of many diseases. Its effectiveness in the prevention and treatment of these diseases, including the flu, has never been scientifically proved to the satisfaction of most scientists.

Q. Does eating garlic or wearing it around your neck protect you from the flu?

A. No, but it will make you noticeable to people near you. Historically, garlic has been widely used as a talisman against many diseases including the flu, bubonic plague and smallpox.

Q. Are overweight people more susceptible to the flu?

A. No, but they are more susceptible to a variety of other diseases such as diabetes mellitus, hypertension and heart disease, so many obese people do turn up in the "high risk" flu category.

CHAPTER II

How the Flu Can Affect You—
Four Case Histories

Influenza A and B are always in the air, causing a few mild cases of flu all year round. Epidemics are different—many more people are affected, and they become much more seriously ill. Epidemics of Influenza A tend to occur every two to four years, at which time a new strain appears on the scene. The severity and the symptoms of the flu vary according to strain. But during a given epidemic, the symptoms tend to be very similar from patient to patient. In some epidemics, such as the one in 1939, insomnia and dizziness commonly occurred. In 1968, many patients experienced ringing in the ears from the Hong Kong flu virus. The Port Chalmers Influenza A virus, which caused epidemics in 1974 and 1975, made many patients sleepy, even weeks after they had recovered.

Because there are so many strains of the Influenza A virus, the flu appears to have many faces. The development of complications adds a dimension to the ordinary pattern of the disease. Taking all of the recent outbreaks as a composite, certain clinical patterns can be seen. There are cases of mild influenza, moderately severe influenza, moderately severe influenza complicated by bacterial pneumonia, and severe influenza complicated by influenza pneumonia. In order to best describe these forms of the disease, I am going to share with you some illustrative case histories.

Case 1. Mild Influenza

John Chaffee was a nineteen-year-old college student in his second year of premedical studies at UCLA. Late on Wednesday afternoon, as he put the finishing touches on an article for the campus paper, he began to feel aches and pains all over his body. From his small desk in the crowded newspaper office he looked out into the bleak November day hanging over Los Angeles. It had been a cold day, cloudy and damp, and now he recalled that he had even felt a bit chilly in his calculus class at mid-morning.

"Gee, I feel lousy," he said to another student editor, Frank Alejo.

"What's the matter?"

"My whole body aches. I feel like I want to lie down and die."

"You don't look sick," said Frank, a bit skeptically.

"Maybe I don't, but I'm certainly coming down with something."

Standing up didn't make John feel any better, nor did stretching his arms and legs and twisting his body. "I think I'd better go home."

"Can you drive all right?" asked Frank.

"I think so."

The cold air made him feel worse, and once inside the car he began having terrible chills, in spite of the hot air pouring out of the heater. It was only a twenty-minute drive to his house, but it seemed like an eternity. He didn't think he would make it.

His mother was reading a newspaper when he walked through the back door. She only had to take one look at him.

"You look terrible!" she exclaimed. "What's the matter?"

John didn't have the strength to answer. He just nodded his head and shuffled into the dining room, limply placing his coat on a chair and his books on the table. Now that he was home, an intense craving to lie down in bed had come over him.

"Oh, you must be getting the flu," he heard his mother say as he dragged himself upstairs. "I heard on the radio there's a big epidemic on the way, from New York."

Lying down in bed didn't help. He tossed and turned, trying to find a comfortable position. His father came up to see him, felt his forehead and said to his wife, "He has a high fever." When they took his temperature, the thermometer read 103.6° Fahrenheit. John felt his body burning up, but his feet were cold as ice. His parents forced him to take some aspirin and orange juice. The orange juice had no taste at all and the thought of food nauseated him.

John spent an unpleasant, feverish night, tossing and turning with body aches and nightmares. The next morning was as bleak as the day before, and if anything he felt worse. At 9 A.M. his temperature was 101.4° F. During the night he had developed a cough and a sore throat and running nose.

"How do you feel?" asked his mother, holding out a glass of orange juice and two aspirins.

"The same," came John's reluctant reply. But there was one small improvement: at least he could taste the orange juice now.

Dr. Sidney Kalish had been the Chaffees' family physician ever since they had moved to Baldwin fifteen years before. When he arrived at 11 A.M. he had already heard John's story from Mr. Chaffee over the phone.

"It looks like you have the flu," he said with a bit of a smile. John tried to muster a smile between coughing and putting a facial tissue to his nose to stop the dripping. Dr. Kalish looked down John's throat and into his ears, felt his neck and put his stethoscope to his chest. He took his temperature. It had risen from the earlier low of 101.4° to 102.2°.

"Well, it's nothing but the flu," he said, closing his black bag. John had drifted back into his pillow and Dr. Kalish spoke more to his mother than to him. "I want him to stay in bed for the next couple of days. Give him plenty of fluids, and two aspirin every four hours, and start him on soup and a bland diet."

"Doesn't he need an antibiotic?" John heard his mother's question only dimly. His ears were stuffed up and ringing.

"No, he's young and strong. He'll recover nicely in a couple of days. O.K. John," he said, "remember, stay in bed." John nodded feebly. The way he felt, he couldn't imagine himself ever getting up out of bed again.

"Is there a lot of flu around, Doctor?" asked Mrs. Chaffee as the two of them went down the stairs together.

"Oh, yes," said Dr. Kalish. "There is quite an epidemic going on because of this Hong Kong virus."

By dinner time John's temperature was down to 99.8° and the aches and pains were less severe. He had enough of an appetite to eat some soup and drink some juice. On Friday morning the aches and pains disappeared and he felt much better.

"I feel like I've been beaten up," he said to his mother as she brought him some toast and juice. He steadily improved and by the fifth day of his illness was able to get up out of bed. His temperature was normal, but he had a cough and a thick nasal discharge. John was able to return to classes on Monday morning. "I still feel washed out," he said as he met his friend Frank in the hall. It took another week before he felt his normal self again.

John Chaffee had an uncomplicated bout of the flu. As routine as it was, his parents were right to call in the family physician. The doctor did more than simply confirm what everyone already knew. He was able to ascertain something the Chaffees could not have known—that John was not developing any of the more serious complications of the flu. He was young and in good health and so his physician knew that his chances of rapid recovery without complications were very good. At the end of five days he was able to get out of bed—this is about the average time it takes for an otherwise healthy person to recover from the acute stage. Feeling weak for several days afterward, as John Chaffee did, is also normal.

Case 2. Moderately Severe Influenza

Virginia Rogers was a forty-five-year-old housewife who lived in Springfield, Illinois. She began feeling ill about 10 A.M. on a Friday morning as she started the washing machine down in the basement. "I must be getting a cold," she thought to herself as she climbed up the stairs. She made herself some tea. "It should warm me up," she thought. Outside it was snowing, the kind of snow that falls slowly and clings to the branches of the trees. As she sipped her tea at the kitchen table, she listened to the radio. Kissinger was in Moscow, the civil war in Lebanon was worse, there would be four inches of snow and the flu had come to the city of Springfield.

The tea tasted good, but it didn't make her feel better. She had chills, aches and pains all over, a headache and some dizziness. "I'd better lie down for a while," she said to herself. But that didn't help either. Her nose felt stuffed up and she had a cough.

Billy Rogers, ten years old, came bounding off the school bus and across the snow-covered lawn. "Mom, I'm home," he shouted. There was no response, so he tracked snow down into the basement and finally up the stairs to the main bedroom.

Billy had never seen his mother lying down during the day. "What's the matter, Mom?" he asked, knowing something must be wrong. She knew he was upset, but she really didn't feel like answering him.

"Mom is sick," she said halfheartedly.

"I'll call dad," he said.

"Dad is on his way home," she said quietly.

When John Rogers came home at 5 P.M. Virginia had a fever of 104.6° and a voice so hoarse she could hardly talk. He gave her some aspirin and grapefruit juice and called Dr. Richard Bergson, their family physician. Dr. Bergson was out, so John left a message with the answering service. It was 11 P.M. before the doctor called back. He had been tied up with an emergency. One of his patients, an elderly man, had been shoveling snow and had had a heart attack.

"It sounds like the flu," he said when John Rogers finished describing his wife's condition. "I'll be by first thing in the morning. Keep her in bed, and give her plenty of fluids and aspirin every four hours."

Virginia passed a very bad night. She felt like an oven; her throat ached and no air could get through her nostrils.

Dr. Bergson arrived at 8 A.M. and found that, in addition to the flu, she had a severe laryngitis and bronchitis.

"She has a pretty severe case of the flu," he told John Rogers after they had both gone downstairs. "I want her to stay in bed and drink plenty of fluids."

He went on to explain that she had already developed two complications of the flu—laryngitis and bronchitis—and for that reason he was putting her on an antibiotic.

Virginia's condition remained the same until Monday, except that on Sunday she began coughing up green-yellow sputum. Most of the time her fever hovered around 102.6°. But then on Monday her temperature fell for the first time to 100.2° and by Wednesday it was 99.6°. Dr. Bergson had returned to see her on Monday, but even though her fever was down he advised that she remain in bed. Not until Friday, when she felt much improved, did he allow her to get up out of bed.

Dr. Bergson kept her on the antibiotic for a full ten days. After she got up out of bed, Virginia tired easily for the next two weeks and then gradually regained her strength. A month passed before she felt normal again.

Although Virginia Rogers had only a routine case of the flu, she quickly developed a severe laryngitis and bronchitis. Her husband made the right decision when he heard her hoarse voice and called in the family physician. Dr. Bergson diagnosed her complications early and prevented their developing further, perhaps into pneumonia, by prescribing an antibiotic. If Virginia's husband had adopted a wait-and-see attitude, while treating her with aspirin and fruit juice, he would only have had to wait seven days or so before seeing her develop a serious case of pneumonia. When Virginia began spitting up green-yellow sputum, this meant that in addition to the flu she had a bacterial infection of her respiratory tract. The flu virus itself does not produce sputum of this kind.

The discharges generated by the flu virus are usually clear and watery. Pus-producing bacteria which can complicate ordinary flu infections turn this clear discharge into a yellow-green color.

Virginia was kept on an antibiotic for a full ten days, under her doctor's supervision. Taking antibiotics for only a few days is usually inadequate for the prevention and treatment of complications. Most antibiotics prescribed for flu complications should be taken regularly for a week to ten days.

Case 3. Moderately Severe Influenza Complicated by Bacterial Pneumonia

David Bradley enjoyed his work as a carpenter for a large construction firm in New Orleans. It was February, that time of year when the long rainy season in New Orleans is coming to an end. For the past several months, Dave had been working on a tall office building that was being built at the foot of Canal Street. It was an easy commute to this job since he lived just over the river in Metarie.

One morning Dave and his partner Bill O'Brien were putting up the two-by-fours for a wall on the thirty-second floor.

"Gee, I feel awfully tired," he said to Bill.

"Didn't you get enough sleep?" asked his partner.

"I slept nine hours last night, like a baby."

"Aw, you're just overworked. That foreman has been pushing too hard. For two cents I'd report him to the shop steward."

"Yeah, maybe you're right. I'm probably just a little run down."

By noon, Dave felt pretty bad. He had aches and pains all over his body, a headache and a sore throat. He felt warm, but the chills came and went.

Bill O'Brien knew Dave was no sissy. "I'm gonna take you home," he said. Dave protested, but only weakly. He could hardly stand.

It was as much out of character for Bill O'Brien to be solicitous as for Dave to be sick. But both knew they had no choice. Bill drove Dave home, helped him up to his bedroom and promised to call that evening.

"What could it be?" asked Dave.

"Darned if I know," said his wife Ginny, "but some hot tea and soup will fix you up in no time." Ginny Bradley had raised six children, and sickness was no stranger to her. Raised on a farm in northern Louisiana, the oldest of ten brothers and sisters, she had seen plenty of sickness even before she married Dave. She knew just what to do.

Dave had no appetite, so the tea and soup went down painfully. Ginny took his temperature. It was 103.6°. By early afternoon he had a cough and his voice became hoarse.

The Bradley house was no place to be sick in. There were four boys still at home, ranging from ten to seventeen. The living room often substituted as a football field, pop music filled one upstairs bedroom and trombone practice went on in the playroom.

In spite of aspirin, juice and soup, Dave felt more and more miserable. When Bill asked over the phone that evening, "How's he doing?" he expected some good news. Instead, Ginny told him that Dave was worse.

"You'd better get a doctor, then," advised Bill.

Getting a doctor to make house calls in New Orleans was not easy. Physicians tried to avoid it, not only because it was time-consuming, but because they'd found that carrying a black bag increased their chances of being mugged.

Dr. Philip De Marco was the Bradleys' family physician. But when Ginny called him the answering service operator said, "Dr. De Marco is out of town for a few days. His practice is being covered by Dr. Robert Cohen." Ginny left word with the operator, and around 10 P.M. Dr. Cohen called back.

Ginny explained Dave's condition. "It sounds like the flu," said Dr. Cohen. "Just keep him in bed and give him plenty of aspirin and fluids. Bring him over to my office at 11 A.M. tomorrow."

Ginny was too timid to ask Dr. Cohen, whom she had never met, to come to the house. She hoped Dave would improve by morning. Dave spent a sleepless night and the next day was so hoarse he could hardly speak. Ginny continued to nurse him as best she could, but he was too sick to be taken to Dr. Cohen's office. Dave spent the next two days at home. If anything, his condition grew worse. He started coughing up green-yellow sputum.

Ginny called Dr. De Marco's office the day he returned from a medical meeting in Baton Rouge. Dr. De Marco did not have to hear the full story to know that Dave was in trouble. He was at the Bradleys' within the hour.

"Hi, Doc," Dave said in his hoarse, weakened voice.

"Ginny here tells me you've been pretty sick." Dave nodded his head slowly.

"Well, let's see what's going on," said Dr. De Marco.

Dave's temperature was 104.6°, rather high for someone in the fifth day of a flu illness. Dr. De Marco examined his throat and found it red and splotched with pus. But the real problem came to light when he listened to Dave's chest with his stethoscope. The unmistakable crackling sounds of pneumonia were present on the right side.

"You've had some pain here, haven't you?" queried the doctor, touching that part of Dave's chest.

"Is it bad?" asked Ginny nervously.

"I'm going to put you in the hospital, Dave. You have not only the flu, but also a lobar pneumonia, and I don't want to take any chances."

It didn't take the ambulance long to get to the Tours Hospital. And within minutes Dave was rushed through the X-ray department and then up to a room on the fourth floor. Ginny and the two oldest boys went to the admitting office to fill out Dave's forms.

They found Dr. De Marco and an intern, Dr. Elizabeth Walker, in Dave's room an hour later. An intravenous had been set up in Dave's left arm.

"We're going to start you on large doses of an antibiotic," said Dr. De Marco as a nurse injected the yellow fluid into the intravenous bottle. "Dr. Walker will check on you from time to time."

The X-rays showed that Dave had a lobar pneumonia. But now tests had to be done to uncover the cause of it. "We have to examine your sputum, Dave, so I want you to cooperate with the nurses. We have to identify the bug causing the pneumonia so we can treat you with the right antibiotic."

It was two days before the test results returned. Dave's condition did not improve in the meantime, which made both doctors suspect that the antibiotic in the intravenous bottle was not killing the germs in Dave's lung.

"Well, it's resistant to ampicillin, Liz," said Dr. De Marco.

"That's why he hasn't improved," nodded Dr. Walker.

The bacteriologic culture of Dave's sputum revealed that a bacterium known as *Staphylococcus aureus* was the cause of his pneumonia. It was resistant to a number of antibiotics but especially sensitive to one.

"We're going to start you on a new antibiotic," said Dr. De Marco. "Within three days you should feel better."

Dr. De Marco's prediction was off by a day, but on the fourth day Dave began to feel better and within a week his chest X-ray showed that the pneumonia was healing. It took another ten days of treatment before Dave was able to return home. He had to recuperate for another two weeks before returning to work. Spring was in full bloom when he returned to join Bill O'Brien, who was now putting up two-by-fours on the thirty-fifth floor.

Dave Bradley started off with a routine case of the flu, but rapidly developed a laryngitis. Had he been vigorously treated with antibiotics at this point, the laryngitis would most likely have cleared. The first mistake was made when neither he nor his wife took the illness seriously. They probably wouldn't have called their family doctor if their friend, Bill O'Brien, had not urged them to. As it turned out, their own doctor was away and the physician covering him was unwilling to make a house call. When Dave was unable to go to the doctor's office, Ginny Bradley should have called another physician or taken Dave to the emergency room of a hospital. She did neither, because she didn't view a case of flu as all that serious.

The third mistake was made when they waited two more days as Dave's condition worsened and he developed a secondary bacterial pneumonia. This probably would not have happened had he been seen earlier by a physician and placed on an appropriate antibiotic.

By the time Dave was admitted to the hospital he had a full-blown bacterial pneumonia. He was treated quickly and efficiently. But in spite of this it took weeks for him to recover. As it turned out, the pneumonia-causing organism was resistant to the first antibiotic used. It is possible that even if he had been placed on an antibiotic earlier, while he was still at home, the organism would have been resistant to it, and the pneumonia might have developed anyway. But, had that occurred, his physician would have been aware of it and could have taken the appropriate measures.

Case 4. Severe Influenza Complicated by Influenza Pneumonia

Mary Evans was twenty years old, a tall, pleasant girl with blond hair and blue eyes. A graduate of Thomas Jefferson High School in Brooklyn, New York, she had been working for a year for an advertising firm on Madison Avenue. She was engaged to Tom McNamara, a fourth-year student at New York University. Tom had been accepted at the Columbia University School of Law for September. He and Mary were planning a June wedding and had already begun apartment hunting, although it was still December.

It was a Tuesday morning when Mary became very ill. She had passed a restless night, but she left for work as usual. She was riding uptown on the crowded Lexington Avenue subway when she began feeling chilly and achy all over. She had to change from the express train to the local at 42nd Street. While waiting for the local she realized that her throat was sore. Then her train arrived, and two minutes later Mary was delivered to her stop at Fifty-first Street. She started to walk toward her office.

It was a clear and cold day with a strong wind blowing down Fifty-third Street. People bucked it as they walked over to Madison Avenue. Mary's office was only a block and a half from the subway, but even so she felt pretty miserable by the time she got there. Her boss, John Shepherd, was a perceptive person and he immediately suspected that she was sick.

"You don't look well, Mary," he said.

"Well, Mr. Shepherd, I really feel pretty bad. It started last night, and forty-five minutes ago, on the way to the office, I began to feel really sick."

Mary and Tom had planned to go Christmas shopping after work. They had made dinner reservations at the Top of the Six's and from there were going to shop along Fifth Avenue.

"I think you ought to go home," advised John Shepherd.

"When Tom calls, could you tell him I'm home?"

"Sure."

Mary went back to her apartment on East Twelfth Street by taxi. She took her temperature. It was 102.6°. She felt chilled and had terrible aches throughout her body. Tom called at noon, after he had called the office and been told that she was ill at home. His classes ended at 4 P.M. and he promised to come right over from the Washington Square campus.

Mary's condition worsened during the afternoon. She developed a cough and generally felt worse. When Tom arrived at 4:30 P.M. he found her in bed. He took her temperature. It was 103.6°. He gave her two aspirins every four hours, but her temperature did not fall. The following morning, Mary felt worse. She had developed a cough and felt some pain on both sides of her chest. She complained to Tom that she was having trouble breathing. He became alarmed and decided to take her to a nearby hospital by ambulance.

The emergency room was crowded, but they took Mary into a cubicle right away.

Dr. Edward Rogers was the intern on duty. He was examining a boy with a minor cut on his leg when a nurse called him over to Mary's cubicle. The nurse had taken Mary's temperature and found it to be 104.3°.

"What seems to be the trouble?" the doctor asked Tom.

"She became sick two days ago," Tom said, and then went on to describe Mary's symptoms. Mary didn't speak. She only nodded yes or no whenever Dr. Rogers asked her questions. He examined her throat, felt her neck for swollen glands and then listened to her chest. "Breathe in and out slowly and deeply," he told her, "with your mouth open." He listened for a long time and then re-listened. Tom grew anxious. Dr. Rogers heard the unmistakable sounds of pneumonia in both lungs.

He took off his stethoscope and helped Mary lie back on the stretcher. Then he motioned Tom outside into the hallway. "I think she has pneumonia," he said.

"How bad is it?" asked Tom.

"I can't say. We'll have to take an X-ray to see."

Mary was wheeled over to the Radiology Department. When the chest film was placed up against the white opaque glass of the viewing box for Dr. Rogers to see, he said, "These viral pneumonias always look worse than they sound." Mary had a bilateral influenza pneumonia, one of the most serious complications of the flu.

She was admitted to the isolation floor by Dr. Robert Geiger, the chief of infectious diseases. He explained to Tom that Mary's condition was very serious, and that for that reason he was placing her on intravenous feedings and intravenous antibiotics. Dr. Geiger had a reputation for being direct, blunt and highly competent. "She has a fifty-fifty chance," he said to Tom. "I can't guarantee anything." Tom was shocked. He had never thought pneumonia was that serious. But Dr. Geiger explained that Mary had a viral pneumonia, the kind which is not affected by antibiotics.

"We are going to give her a drug called amantadine," he explained to Tom. "It can kill the influenza virus if it gets into the body's cells before the virus does." It was an outside chance at best, but worth the try.

In spite of the antibiotic, amantadine, and intravenous fluids, Mary's condition worsened. Late that evening they placed her in an oxygen tent because she had so much difficulty breathing. Tom waited outside the isolation ward all night. There was no change in Mary's condition. By morning she was semi-conscious and her breathing was extremely labored. Tom noticed that her lips were blue. It was all a nightmare to him. Throughout the day, Mary's condition worsened. In spite of heroic efforts, she died at 5 P.M. of massive influenza pneumonia.

Mary Evans caught a routine case of the flu. But eventually she went on to develop one of the rare complications of the flu, an influenza pneumonia, which is often fatal. Tom McNamara did the correct thing when he took her by ambulance to a nearby hospital. The physicians who attended Mary used every modality at their disposal. But in spite of this she died, because there is essentially no specific treatment for influenza pneumonia.

The flu is not a disease that you can shrug off lightly. Although it tends to follow a predictable course in most people, complications can always occur. These complications can usually be prevented or minimized effectively, but not in the case of influenza pneumonia. For this reason, you should not hesitate to get medical help for what you may consider to be a routine case of the flu.

CHAPTER III

How You Can Treat the Flu

The spectacular advances of medical science have not as yet produced an effective drug for curing the flu, but they have confirmed the value of non-specific supportive measures, including some that mothers and grandmothers have advocated probably for centuries. Listed below are some basic facts which you should know about treating the flu.

Q. Does bed rest help to cure the flu?

A. Yes it does. Bed rest is *essential* in treating the flu. It permits your body to rest and enables it to combat the flu infection more effectively.

Q. How useful is plain aspirin in treating the flu?

A. Aspirin is very useful in treating the flu. It reduces fever and alleviates to some extent the body aches and pains so familiar to flu sufferers.

Q. When aspirin does not help the aches and pains of the flu, what else can the patient take?

A. It has been found that small doses of codeine alleviate the body aches and pains caused by the flu. However, codeine has no effect on the fever caused by the flu. It should only be used on the recommendation of a physician and according to his instructions.

Q. Why do physicians advise flu patients to drink plenty of fluids?

A. The high fever caused by the flu causes dehydration and loss of the body's salts and water. Drinking fluids combats this effect of the fever.

Q. What fluids are best in treating the flu?

A. In the early acute phase of the flu most patients lose their appetites, even for fluids. Juices of various kinds are more palatable than any other type of fluid during the acute phase of the flu. They provide the patient with fluid replacement and some sugar and vitamins. Warm soups of a bland.nature should be started as soon as possible, also.

Q. Why is it advisable to eat protein-containing foods when recuperating from the flu?

A. Illnesses like the flu, with their associated fevers, cause a breakdown of body cells. To rebuild the body's cells one needs protein-containing foods.

Q. My twelve-year-old son came down with the flu two days ago and still will not eat solid food. What should I do?

A. Most children regain their appetites by the third or fourth day if they have a moderate case of the flu. In the meantime it is best to give them juices and bland soups. It is unwise to force solid foods on children too soon. If they are still acutely ill with the flu, this will often cause them to vomit.

Q. My husband has been in bed for three days now with the flu. His appetite is beginning to return. What kinds of food should I give him?

A. Flu patients generally do well starting off on a bland diet, which is easily digestible and more palatable to people who've been off their food for a few days. Tea, toast with a little jelly, broiled steak or chicken and boiled vegetables are all good to start with. Light, bland soups are also recommended. They provide some essential nutrients and needed salts.

Q. Is there any truth to the claim that chicken soup helps to cure the flu?

A. Chicken soup has historically been given to patients sick with the flu and other illnesses that produce a high fever, in a number of cultures around the world. It has no specific curative effect. But it is a good supportive measure, since it serves as a palatable food containing some essential nutrients for patients with depressed appetites.

Q. My wife has just come down with the flu. Should I give her some antihistamines to stop her nose from running?

A. Antihistamines are often useful in reducing the degree of nasal discharge in patients with upper respiratory tract infections. However, it is best to use them only under the advice of a physician.

Q. Are over-the-counter cold medicines good for treating the flu?

A. They might afford some temporary relief. But it is not advisable to use them. Most of them contain antihistamines that would suppress a patient's symptoms. While he might welcome the relief, the false impression might be given that he is recovering, when in fact the disease continues to thrive. This would leave him open to possibly serious complications.

Q. Is it a good idea to use a heating pad to relieve chills and to make sure the patient is warm enough?

A. No. Most patients with the flu will find a heating pad uncomfortable anyway.

Q. Do mustard plasters help cure the flu?

A. No, they do not.

Q. How long should one remain in bed when sick with the flu?

A. A good rule of thumb is to remain in bed until the temperature has returned to normal.

Q. What will happen if I get up when I still have a fever?

A. Bed rest lets the body put most of its energy into combating the flu infection. Getting up from bed when you still have a fever weakens your body defenses and makes you more susceptible to complications.

Q. Why do some people get a flu relapse?

A. Often it is not a relapse at all, but a continuation of the same bout of the flu. Patients who get up from bed too soon and start going to work while still feeling feverish, weaken their defenses. The temperature often rises again and forces them to return to bed. Their recuperation is thus prolonged.

Q. What should be done with facial tissues used by flu patients?

A. It is best to have the person put the tissues into a paper bag kept at the bedside and then close the bag and either incinerate it or put it in the garbage can.

Q. My fourteen-year-old son has come down with the flu. Should we let him use the same bathroom as my husband and myself?

A. If you have only one bathroom you have no choice. If you have a spare bathroom it would be preferable to have him use it. In either case, he should be careful to use only his own face towels and bath towels.

Q. Should he use the same tube of toothpaste?

A. No. He should be given a separate tube. Also his toothbrush should be kept separate from those of other family members. Otherwise his infection may spread from his brush to yours.

Q. Should a mother who has the flu take care of her baby?

A. It would be preferable for the husband to do so or to bring in someone. If she has a moderately severe case of the flu, caring for a baby is too much exertion for her. Also, if she does so the risks of passing the infection on to the child are increased.

Q. My daughter is sixteen years old. She has a fever of 99.6° and has been sick with the flu for three days. She wants to wash her hair. Should I allow her to?

A. No. It is best not to allow her to until her fever goes all the way down to normal.

Q. Should people with the flu takes baths and showers?

A. Most people with a high temperature have no desire to take a shower or bath. It is best to wait until the temperature gets down to normal before doing so. A sponge bath can, however, be taken in bed.

Q. Is it necessary to call a physician if I'm sure it's just the flu?

A. Yes. It is always best to contact your physician even if you are sure you have the flu. The flu can be a serious disease, and complications like laryngitis and pneumonia develop fairly rapidly. Such complications can often be prevented or effectively treated with appropriate medications.

Q. I have two sons, twelve and ten. They share a bedroom. The older just came down with the flu. Should I have the ten-year-old use another room?

A. Yes. Although he may have already contracted the flu from his brother, you will reduce his chances of getting it if you put him in another room.

Q. Does hot tea cure the flu?

A. Hot tea is a good beverage for flu patients if they like it. It has no direct curing effect, but it is a good supportive measure.

Q. Two of my children are sick with the flu. Should I disinfect their pajamas and bed linen before washing them?

A. No, this is not necessary. Washing them in hot water is sufficient.

Q. My nineteen-year-old son has the flu. Should I wash my hands after going into his room to bring him his food and take his temperature?

A. Yes. Hand-washing is essential in the management of flu cases and should be impressed on all family members.

Q. Is it unsafe to touch your face while in the same room with a flu patient?

A. Although one risks contracting the flu just by being in the same room as a flu patient, touching one's face does increase that risk.

Q. How often should one change the bedding and clothing of a flu patient?

A. These should be changed every day and laundered right away.

Q. My husband has the flu and has been sleeping on and off for about twelve hours a day. Is this harmful? Should I wake him periodically or let him sleep?

A. This is not harmful and you should not wake him. Many flu patients sleep more hours than they normally do. If you are worried about this, consult your doctor.

Q. My ten-year-old son has the flu. Some of his friends want to visit him. Should I let them?

A. No. Your son could pass the infection on to them.

Q. I have heard that there are certain drugs called antiviral agents which can be used for treating the flu. Is there any truth to this?

A. There is a drug called amantadine which is effective against the influenza viruses. However, for it to be effective, it must be given before the virus enters the body's cells. By the time the first symptoms of the flu appear, the virus is already inside of the body's cells and thus amantadine is of no use. Another problem with this drug is that it has serious side effects. For these reasons it has not proved very effective in treating the flu. There is no other drug useful in treating the flu.

Q. Does liquor speed up recovery from the flu?

A. No, it does not.

Q. Is sitting up in bed harmful if you are ill with the flu?

A. No.

Q. If I'm sick with the flu, how often can I get up out of bed?

A. It is best to only get out of bed to go to the bathroom. Once your body temperature returns to normal, you can get up and begin to resume normal activity.

Q. How long should I stay at home if I get the flu?

A. Bed rest is recommended for at least as long as you have a fever. If you feel strong enough, you can go out, weather permitting, when your temperature has been normal for a day.

Q. If I get the flu do I need to have a chest X-ray?

A. Only if your physician recommends it after examining you.

Q. Can the flu lead to water on the lung?

A. "Water on the lung" is a popular term for a pleural effusion, a fluid accumulation in the pleural cavity in which the lungs are located. A pleural effusion can occur as a complication of the flu. The first sign that you might be developing one is a pain in your chest—a sharper, more localized pain than the general achiness of the flu. If you experience any pain like this, call your doctor immediately.

Q. Is smoking bad for you if you are sick with the flu?

A. If you have the flu, don't smoke. It predisposes you to complications.

Q. Do liniments rubbed on the chest help cure the flu?

A. No, they have no direct curative effect.

Q. Does it help to keep taking Vitamin C after you've come down with the flu?

A. As I mentioned earlier, there is no medical consensus on the effectiveness of Vitamin C in treating respiratory ailments. But taking Vitamin C does seem a reasonable, probably effective way of helping your body recover after a bout of the flu.

Q. What steps should I take if I think I have the flu?

A. 1. Go to bed.
  2. Call your family physician.
  3. Follow his advice. He will want you to get plenty of bed rest, take aspirin every four hours and drink a lot of fluids.
  4. When your appetite returns, don't push it. Start on a bland diet.
  5. Contact your doctor if: your voice becomes hoarse, you develop pains in your chest, you have difficulty breathing, or you start bringing up yellow- or green-colored phlegm.
  6. Take whatever medications your doctor advises.
  7. Stay in bed until your temperature returns to normal.
  8. Remain at home for at least one day after your temperature has been normal.
  9. Resume your regular activities gradually.

Q. What should I do if my doctor cannot make a house call and cannot see me in his office for a week or more?

A. It is unlikely that these two situations would occur simultaneously. Some physicians who are not able to see a patient immediately either at home or in the office can evaluate the patient's condition by obtaining a history over the phone. They can then prescribe a course of treatment. If you are unable to obtain even this minimal level of care you should call another physician. If you can't make contact with another doctor, go to the emergency room of a nearby hospital. Do not be embarrassed to take your own case seriously. Flu is usually not a severe disease, but it can be if not treated promptly and properly.

Q. How should I evaluate my symptoms if my doctor is too busy to see me or cannot come to my home?

A. Evaluating your own symptoms can be dangerous. You should not do it. If you cannot make even telephone contact with your doctor, you should call another physician.

Q. What should I tell my doctor over the phone when I speak with him?

A. Your doctor will ask the right questions. He will ask you, When did you become sick? Do you have a fever? Do you have a sore throat? Do you have body aches and pains? Have you had chills? Have you had nausea, vomiting or diarrhea? Have you lost your appetite? Are you coughing? If so, are you bringing up any phlegm? What color is it? Do you have any pains in your chest? Judging by your answers, and by evaluating the sound of your voice, your doctor will be able to arrive at a tentative decision about your condition.

Q. What steps can I take to keep the flu from developing into pneumonia?

A. Early and correct treatment of the flu—which means bed rest, adequate fluid intake and proper nutrition—under the guidance of your doctor, who may prescribe antibiotics if he thinks they are called for, are the best steps you can take to prevent the development of pneumonia. Only a small proportion of flu victims develop pneumonia. Cases most often occur among high-risk people such as those with chronic lung and heart problems. Their best defense against the flu and potential pneumonia is early vaccination with flu vaccine. If they get the flu they should be put on antibiotics by their physicians to help prevent the development of pneumonia.

Q. What are the first signs of pneumonia?

A. Pneumonia can be caused by a number of different microorganisms. The bacterial pneumonias that complicate the flu often start with abrupt chills, fever, breathing difficulty, coughing and pain in the chest. These symptoms occur a few days after the start of the flu. You should not try to evaluate these symptoms yourself. Consult your family doctor.

Q. What are the symptoms of pneumonia in children?

A. Symptoms vary, depending on which microorganism is responsible for the pneumonia. In infants and young children from four to eighteen months of age, the influenza virus occasionally causes a form of pneumonia known as bronchiolitis. Most cases of bronchiolitis are due to other types of viruses, however. The symptoms start with wheezing and difficult breathing, and a staccato cough which may be constant. Within two or three days, breathing becomes more difficult and the child may become cyanotic—that is, his skin will turn bluish, indicating a lack of oxygen in the blood.

Pneumonias due to bacteria present a variety of symptoms, including high fever, chills, restlessness, pain in the chest, difficult breathing and a hacking cough. In small children, febrile convulsions may occur. Some children may also develop vomiting and diarrhea. There is considerable variation in the combination and severity of symptoms from one child to another. Keep track of how your child feels. If you have any doubts about his condition, call your doctor.

As you can see, you *can* fight back against the flu. It is not—as many people believe—a disease that must simply be left to take its course. You can alter its course for the better, shorten it, and avoid major complications by doing everything within your own power to treat yourself, and by following the advice of your physician.

Part Two

MANKIND
VERSUS THE FLU

CHAPTER IV

A Quick History of the Flu

The flu is certainly no stranger to the human race, although it is difficult to say just how long the disease has been around. No doubt many of the so-called plagues referred to by ancient writers were actually flu epidemics. But they are so poorly described that medical historians cannot safely include them in the history of the flu.

The reliable records that do exist indicate that the flu occurred as an epidemic disease every few years in various parts of Europe and the rest of the world. "Epidemic" means that many people in a local area became ill over a relatively short period of time. At longer intervals—every thirty years or so—pandemics occurred. "Pandemic" means that many people in many countries all over the world became ill. This is still the pattern of flu today.

The first clearly-described flu pandemic occurred in 1173 in Italy, Germany, France and England. In 1357, the disease was first called *influenza,* which is now its scientific name. It came from the Italian word meaning "influence," since the appearance of the disease was believed to be influenced by the stars. But although the word influenza was coined in the Middle Ages when astrological attributions for diseases were common, it did not come into popular usage until the eighteenth century.

Unlike many medieval diseases, the flu disappeared for decades at a time. Smallpox, typhus, typhoid fever and other contagious diseases were always around and people never forgot them. But once a flu pandemic was over, they tended to forget about it. Knowledge of previous flu pandemics was often lost, since information had to be transferred orally from one generation to the next. For this reason, a pandemic was often viewed as a brand-new disease, and each one gave rise to a new name for the flu. From the facetious names given to the flu, it is clear that pandemics often caused only mild illness.

In the sixteenth century some English writers referred to it as "the new acquaintance," and "the gentle correction." In the seventeenth century, the English called it "the new delight" and "the jolly rant." Horace Walpole later referred to it as "these blue plagues." Around this period, the French coined the word "la grippe," which is still used today both in French and English. In 1782, the word "influenza" was imported from Italy and became popular in England.

Often the disease was described by a name indicating the country where it was supposed to have originated. Thus the English called it "the French disease," the French, "the English disease," and so forth. The flu was not feared as greatly as some of the other diseases then present in Europe and elsewhere. The Black Death, known scientifically as the bubonic plague, killed nine out of every ten people who contracted it during the Dark Ages. In comparison, only two flu victims in a hundred died in many of these pandemics. So, while almost everyone got it, most recovered, which at that time was reason enough for people to view it with a bit of humor.

One of the best-documented influenza pandemics occurred in Europe in 1510. Although the symptoms of the flu could have been due to other viruses, the characteristics of that epidemic as recorded by several writers leave no doubt that it was the flu. Only the flu could have appeared so suddenly, affected such large numbers of people, both rich and poor, in a short time, and then disappeared. During the sixteenth century the disease was also recorded in Africa and Asia.

Confusing the picture somewhat was the appearance in 1485 of a disease which came to be known as "the sweating sickness" or "the English sweat." It first descended on London right after the end of the War of the Roses. It raged through London for five weeks and took a high mortality among the rich and poor, the young and old. Two lord mayors died and Henry VII had to postpone his coronation at Westminster Abbey. A physician of the day described the disease's symptoms like this:

> ". . . when a grete sweyting and stynking, with redness of the face and of all the body, and a contynual thurst, with a grete headache because of the fumes and venoms . . ."

This disease struck London again in 1507 and a third time in 1517, when Cardinal Wolsey contracted it three times. It reappeared in 1528, and in 1529 it traveled to Germany where Catholics regarded it as punishment from God for Martin Luther's heresies. But only the English seem to have suffered dramatic and sudden symptoms. It became a popular belief that to prevent the disease people had to sweat for at least twenty-four hours without stop. So healthy people who wanted immunity were put to bed and covered with furs and featherbeds. Their beds were placed in rooms where all windows and doors were shut tight and stoves were heated to raise the temperature in the rooms.

In 1844, J.F.K. Hecker, a German medical historian, described the unfortunate results of this practice:

> ". . . in order to prevent the sufferer, should he be somewhat impatient, from throwing off his hot load, some persons in health likewise lay upon him, and thus oppressed him to such a degree, that he could neither stir hand nor foot, and finally in this rehearsal of hell, being bathed in an agonizing sweat, gave up the ghost, when, perhaps, if his too officious relatives had manifested a little discretion, he might have been saved without difficulty."

Such medical practices were not uncommon during the Renaissance, being founded on the theory that producing the symptoms of the disease in a healthy person would immunize him. The high mortality from this particular practice, however, prompted people to modify it, and so when the disease next struck, people were merely sewn up into bags made from bedcovers. Sleep was thought to be dangerous, so a variety of techniques were devised to keep people awake for twenty-four hours, including pulling their hair out and dropping vinegar into their eyes.

There is considerable debate even today whether or not the "English sweat" was really the flu. Many authorities think it was, and point out that the same illness occurred simultaneously in other European countries where it was considered to be the flu. But the suddenness and the violence of the symptoms are perplexing, since they do not fit the usual pattern of the flu.

Medical historian Hecker speculated that it was the flu, and attributed the spectacular symptoms to the English habits of dressing too warmly, taking too many hot baths, using too little soap, being influenced in their personal habits by the high price of linen and, finally, of just being English!

In 1562, a flu epidemic hit Edinburgh, Scotland. Mary Stuart, Scotland's most famous queen, fell victim, as described in this historical account:

> "Immediately upon the Queene's arrival here she fell acquainted with a new disease that is common in this towne, called here the newe acquayntance, which passed throughe her whole courte, neither sparinge lordes, ladyes nor damaysells, nor so much as either French or English. It is a plague in their heades that have yt with a great cough that remayneth with some longer, with others shorter tyme as yt findeth apte bodies for the nature of the disease. The Queene kept her bed six days. There was no appearance of danger, nor manie that die of the disease except some olde folks."

This description, written by a lay observer over four hundred years ago, is a fairly good account of the flu as we know it today.

Some of the medical writings of the period supplement such lay descriptions with good detail which has enabled medical historians to piece together not only the history of the flu but its symptoms, which have not changed in centuries. Even in the sixteenth century the disease caused its greatest mortality among the old and the sick.

Between the twelfth and nineteenth centuries there were probably fourteen pandemics and perhaps eighty epidemics in Europe alone. In Europe and America in the nineteenth century, there were five recognized pandemics, in 1830, 1847–1848, 1857, 1874 and 1889–1890. Of these five, the pandemics of 1847–1848 and 1889–1890 were the most severe and widespread. In England in 1847, five thousand deaths, mostly among the aged, were attributed to the flu. The epidemic lasted for six weeks, and during this period the daily obituary column of *The Times* of London more than tripled. The disease affected all social strata: unlike so many other contagious diseases, the flu traversed the hygienic barriers which usually protected the upper levels of European society.

Then in 1889, after two relatively mild pandemics, the flu appeared again in Asia and Europe. Unlike previous pandemics recorded in England, this one came in four waves, of which the first was fairly mild. It ended in February of 1890 and was followed by a more severe wave in May 1891, a third wave in January 1892 and a fourth in December 1893. The second and third waves each resulted in more than two thousand deaths in London. On January 8, 1892, the Duke of Clarence, eldest son of the Prince of Wales (later Edward VII) and older brother of the future King George V, died of influenza at Sandringham. The succession to the Crown of St. Edward was thus altered by the flu.

The flu did not disappear after 1893. Following a pattern by then observed for over a hundred years, it continued to occur in outbreaks and localized epidemics in 1895, 1900 and 1908. Then came 1918.

The influenza pandemic of 1918–1919 is regarded as one of the greatest human catastrophes of all time. Historians have ranked it with the Plague of Justinian—bubonic plague—which in 542 A.D. killed several million people in Byzantium, and with the Black Death, also bubonic plague, which killed about 25 million people in Europe during the Dark Ages. There were about two billion people living on the earth in 1918 and it is estimated that half of them fell ill with the flu. Of the billion who fell ill, some 22 million are thought to have died. There were 20 million flu cases in the United States alone, by best estimates, and 548,452 deaths. Not since the Black Death, centuries before, had such a catastrophe occurred.

Where did it start? No one is really sure, because milder forms of influenza were present at the time in many distant parts of the world. Although it was called the Spanish influenza in the United States, the evidence shows that it was in the United States for quite a while before it even got to Spain. In Japan the disease was called American influenza, and in China, Japanese influenza; but the term Spanish influenza became accepted as its name all over the world.

In 1918 the world was preoccupied with World War I. The Czar had fallen in Russia, Germany was disintegrating and the Allies were pressing hard on the Western front. The United States Army had grown from its normal peacetime level of 190,000 men to more than 2,000,000, most of them raw recruits from rural America. There was an enormous movement of men across the North American continent, and they were being excessively crowded into hastily built army camps. The trans-Atlantic sea lanes bustled with troop ships whose decks were packed with soldiers sent to bolster the American Expeditionary Force.

No one was really prepared for what eventually happened. But the war mobilization already in progress represented a tremendous asset in dealing with the pandemic. The war had created an atmosphere in which everyone pitched in to do his share. Had the flu struck at a different period, the United States and her allies could not have coped so well with the medical, social, economic and political consequences of the Spanish influenza.

There had been quite a bit of influenza in the United States in

1915 and 1916 as well as in many parts of Europe. But it was the usual kind of flu, relatively mild, incapacitating people for several days and causing only a few deaths. This pattern continued into early 1918. During the months of March and April, three waves of influenza passed through Camp Funston, out on the Kansas prairie. Camp Funston was a huge military reservation, hastily spawned by the necessities of World War I. The barracks were crowded, water supplies were of questionable quality and latrines were lacking. The Chief Medical Officer of Camp Funston was Colonel Edward R. Schreiner, a forty-five-year-old surgeon. He often passed sleepless nights worrying about all the diseases that could break out among the twenty-six thousand men in the camp. The Surgeon General, William C. Gorgas, then a white-haired veteran of public health crusades, had complained of the terribly crowded conditions in Army camps across the country. He had recommended in testimony before a Senate committee that the mobilization of men be put off for a few months until better Army camps were built. But military planners could not wait that long, so more men were recruited and sent into already-crowded camps.

Camp Funston had a large hospital of over three thousand beds, most of which were always filled. There had already been epidemics of measles, mumps, pneumonia and colds, and over two hundred cases of cerebro-spinal meningitis. The hospital had little to offer except nursing care. It was an uncomfortable jumble of brick buildings and wooden barracks.

On March 11, 1918, an Army cook, Albert Gitchell, came to the hospital at 6 A.M. complaining of a cold. His symptoms included sore throat, fever, headache and body aches. A few minutes later a second man appeared, complaining of the same symptoms. By noon Colonel Schreiner had admitted 107 men to the hospital with influenza. By the end of the week there were 522 cases, and at the end of five weeks 1127 cases and 46 deaths. Similar outbreaks occurred in Camp Kearny in California, Camp Johnston in Florida, Camp Lee in Virginia, Camp McClellan in Alabama and Camp Oglethorpe in Georgia. The disease broke out in colleges and prisons and in the general population. In San Quentin five hundred of the two thousand prisoners came down with the flu and three died in April and May.

Outbreaks of this kind were reported all over Europe. In general, the illness was not severe and the mortality was low. French troops came down with it at Tours and Bordeaux, and the Royal Navy registered over ten thousand cases. This first wave of the pandemic was mild.

By August, the picture began to change. The flu was in China and Africa and was looking more ominous. Although the illness was about the same as the one which had occurred in the spring, some patients were suddenly developing a severe pneumonia. Often this occurred just as a person was beginning to feel better: within hours the lips and ears turned a dark purple color and the face became pale. This sequence had only to occur for several weeks before it was recognized by doctors as ultimately fatal. No one knew the reason for this sinister turn of events. Those who had viewed the flu as only a nuisance now looked on it with dread. People with ordinary, mild cases suddenly turned blue and died.

Physicians and scientists all over the world were perplexed. According to Dr. Herbert French of London, autopsies of flu victims revealed that the lungs were "invariably heavier than normal and often greatly so, the increased weight being a feature of the lower lobes rather than the upper. . . . the lung lesions, complex or variable, struck one as being quite different in character from anything one had met with at all. . . ."

Many theories were advanced as to why this flu was so virulent, and a frantic search went on for the microorganism causing it. Viruses had not yet been discovered, so the microscopes of the day revealed conflicting evidence that incriminated a wide assortment of bacteria. In New York City, for example, Dr. William Park, director of the Health Department's laboratories, reported that he had isolated six different bacteria from six members of the same family ill with the flu. It would be another fifteen years before the discovery of the influenza virus.

Many attributed this virulent flu to malnutrition, including Dr. Royal Copeland, the flamboyant Commissioner of Health of New York City. "You haven't heard of our doughboys getting it, have you? You bet you haven't, and you won't," he said on August 14 at a press conference. Dr. Copeland's distinguished appearance was not matched by his public health abilities. A noted ophthalmologist, he was nonetheless more politician than physician. After he stepped down as Commissioner of Health in 1923, he won election to the United States Senate, where he was better known for his long-winded speeches than for his wisdom. Today his photograph hangs on the wall of the boardroom of the New York City Health Department along with those of the commissioners who both preceded and succeeded him.

Dr. Copeland's off-the-cuff witticisms became commonplace in New York City's newspapers. In the late summer the *New York Times* ran the headline "City Is Not in Danger from Spanish Grip," citing Copeland as its source. The article, however, went on to say that "the Commissioner did advise that any fellow kissing a girl would be wiser to do it through a handkerchief." Fortunately for the City of New York, the Department of Health was the finest in the country, with a professional staff which read like a *Who's Who* in public health.

On a warm August morning, the Norwegian liner *Bergensfjord* steamed through New York's lower bay and docked just above the Narrows at the U.S. Army base pier in Brooklyn. Following a procedure set up a short while before at most East Coast ports, the ship was fumigated. The *Bergensfjord*'s journey to New York had been a horror for her passengers. Over a hundred passengers had fallen ill with the flu while in mid-Atlantic, and four had died. The captain, in an attempt to destroy the infection, had the crew wash the decks down with a pungent concoction of ammonia and creosote. The corridors and the rooms were sprayed with an aerosol of the same product, making everyone sick. When the ship docked eleven passengers were seriously ill. Ambulances carried them swiftly from the dock to the Norwegian Hospital. One of them, Mrs. J. Olsen, died a few hours later, becoming the first known person to die of the Spanish influenza in New York City. She had been on her way from Norway to Flint, Michigan to join her husband.

Under the then-existing regulations, it was impossible for either New York City's Health Commissioner or the Surgeon General of the United States Public Health Service—then Dr. Rupert Blue— to prevent the *Bergensfjord* from docking and her passengers from disembarking. Even if they had been empowered to do so, it is unlikely that the flu could have been kept out of the city.

Twenty-seven years had passed since the last flu epidemic had hit New York City. It had been a mild epidemic with few deaths, but that was little comfort to a frightened public that was already fully aware of what was happening all over Europe. The influenza epidemic started in New York City around September 15, 1918 and lasted until November 17. On September 15 a thirty-two-year-old man died of the disease, the first native New Yorker known to have died in the epidemic. By September 30 the daily number of deaths had risen to 48. It continued to rise—89 on October 5, 240 on October 10, 364 on October 16 and then 457 on October 20. Thereafter the number of people who died each day gradually fell, to 456 on October 25, 311 on October 29, 180 on November 5 and 52 on November 16.

New York City's experience was mirrored all over the country. While the epidemic was reaching its peak in New York during the third week of October, the first cases were appearing in New Orleans, Los Angeles and San Francisco. Frantic public health officials fired out bulletins of advice to the public, not knowing what would really work. The United States Public Health Service requested and received a million dollars from Congress to help deal with the desperate situation. All over the country, the flu was killing healthy young adults in the age group fifteen to forty. This had never happened before during flu epidemics. Volunteers were mobilized to visit the sick, care for orphaned children and feed families where everyone was down with the disease. On October 7, the Army rescinded its draft call to 142,000 men, and in the Argonne Forest 16,000 doughboys were sick with what they called "the Spanish lady."

Even the mighty fell victim: Kaiser Wilhelm; King George V; King Alfonso XIII; Prince Max of Baden, chancellor of Germany; and Franklin D. Roosevelt, then Assistant Secretary of the Navy. Mary Pickford was ill in Beverly Hills, British Prime Minister David Lloyd George in Manchester, and Queen Alexandria in Copenhagen.

All over the world new ordinances went into effect in an attempt to stop the flu. Strong efforts were made to curtail the widespread habit of spitting. In New York City, Dr. Royal Copeland called for "spitless Sundays," but his plea had no effect. Dr. Herman Biggs, then Commissioner of Health of New York State, issued a sterner ordinance. A severe fine was levied against anyone who coughed or sneezed in public without covering his or her face with a handkerchief. Huge signs were posted along New York City's streets proclaiming, "It Is Unlawful to Cough and Sneeze." Violators were subject to a fine of five hundred dollars or a year in jail. By the end of the first week, several hundred New Yorkers were arrested. In Chicago, Dr. John Robertson, Commissioner of Health, gave orders to arrest thousands in order to stop people from sneezing in public.

On October 19 San Francisco required that barbers wear face masks, and on October 22 Mayor James Ralph encouraged everyone to wear them. In Sydney, Australia, Shanghai, China, Calgary, Alberta and many other parts of the world, face masks appeared by the thousands. Their proponents argued their cause by citing favorable statistics. Where masks were worn, the number of flu cases was far lower than in areas where they were not worn. Those who opposed the wearing of face masks pointed out flaws in the statistical data. Ingenuity in mask design and decoration was rewarded in some locales with prizes. In Rockford, Illinois, people embroidered skulls and crossbones on their masks. In retrospect, it can be concluded that the wearing of masks did nothing to stop the epidemic. In China it was adopted as a custom by medical personnel who wear masks to this day, even in situations where they are obviously not warranted.

Dr. Royal Copeland, like many other public health officials, tried to minimize the extent of the epidemic in order to allay public fears. He continued to call the epidemic "widespread" and refused to term it "serious," even on a day when 3,096 cases and 364 deaths were recorded. He kept New York City's theaters open, although many had to close anyway because so many of the stage-hands and performers were out sick. "I'm keeping my theaters in as good condition as my wife keeps my home," he told the *New York Times* as the epidemic ran wild.

New York City Mayor John ("Red Mike") Hylan ordered squads of sanitation workers out to the cemeteries in Queens and Brooklyn to dig trenches in which to bury the dead. In some cities, the supply of coffins was rapidly exhausted. A corpse was wrapped in sheets, placed in a coffin and carried to the grave, where it was removed from the coffin and buried. The same coffin was then used again and again to transport other bodies.

The sick crowded hospitals to the point where they had to be bedded down in the halls on the floor. Basic human services were crippled. All over the country schools, churches, theaters, saloons and even public telephone booths were closed down. But in New York City Dr. Royal Copeland decided not to close the schools. This decision was viewed, even at the time, as reckless and not out of character for the blundering, outspoken Commissioner. As soon as he announced it, an avalanche of criticism fell on his head from every quarter. But he stood firm and did not reconsider even when the *New York Times* attacked him. As it turned out, this decision was among the best of his short career as Commissioner of Health.

In October, he met with Dr. S. Josephine Baker, then director of the Department of Health's Bureau of Child Hygiene, a position she had held since 1908. Dr. Baker was a renowned specialist in child health, the author of several books on the subject and an activist for women's rights. More than a half-century later, she is still regarded as a giant in public health and a leading pioneer in the field of public health pediatrics. True to form, Copeland, with much bluff, told her to close down all the schools. And, equally true to form, Dr. Baker, impeccably attired in her man-tailored suit and matching tie, said no. Dr. Copeland was no match for Dr. Baker and was smart enough both to follow her advice and to take public credit for it. He followed her plan, now permanently recorded in the annual report of the Department of Health for 1918. Dr. Baker had her staff of nurses and inspectors visit one-fifth of the 800,000 children who were then in New York City's schools each morning. In addition, the number of children in attendance and the number of absentees were ascertained and telephoned daily to her office. The names and addresses of all absentees were obtained by the medical inspectors and nurses, who then visited the children at home to find out why they were out of school. In this way, outbreaks of flu in families were uncovered and volunteers sent in to care for children whose mothers were laid up. This masterful plan enabled Dr. Baker's staff to continuously monitor the health of New York City's school children and see to it that they and their families were properly cared for when the flu struck. As Dr. Baker knew from her many years of experience amid the squalor of the Lower East Side and Hell's Kitchen, children from these areas were in a healthier environment in school than at home.

Copeland's announcement of this plan drew criticism from people like John Wanamaker and William Randolph Hearst. But he knew Dr. Baker had to be right. And she was. There were very few cases of the flu among New York City's school children. Eventually other cities followed New York's example.

The epidemic overwhelmed the New York City Department of

Health and other such departments all across the country. Beneath the terse, official summary of the department's work that year lies an untold story of human suffering and professional dedication.

> . . . The epidemic of influenza and pneumonia came upon us with an overwhelming force . . . a number of medical and clerical staff deserve special commendation because of the meritorious and unselfish part they played during the trying ordeal when the epidemic was at its height. The nurses and others who labored untiringly on Sundays, holidays and evenings, without added recompense, were always ready to respond to the innumerable calls made upon them.

There was much misery and sorrow, some of it remembered even today by those who either lived through those terrible days or were told about them. The story I know best is the one that involves my own family. It was first told to me thirty years after the siege, but to my grandmother it was still a vivid and horrible memory.

Vincent Insanté was my maternal grandfather. He was born in 1872 in Philppeville, Algeria, now called Skikda, not long after the French consolidated their administrative control over this part of Africa. As a boy growing up in Algeria he had the advantages of being a colonial's son. But he also had to survive diphtheria, typhoid fever, typhus and malaria. After his father perished on a French government expedition to the East African Somali coast, he married an Italian woman who came from the island of Ischia, near Capri. Together they came to the United States and stayed for a while in New York, in Providence, and in Canton, Ohio. After my mother was born, my grandparents returned to Ischia, leaving my mother behind with my grandfather's sister in Ohio.

The Spanish influenza struck their part of Europe in September, but, because Ischia is an island, the disease did not arrive there until October. On November 4, 1918, my grandparents' oldest son, Anthony, came down with the flu. The disease appeared to be fairly mild, but late in the evening of November 10, the boy, who was eight years old, began having trouble breathing. By morning, his condition was worse. There was no hospital on the island and the nearest one was in Naples, four hours away by boat. My grandfather decided to take him there. At sunrise my grandmother accompanied them from the house to the pier in an open horse-drawn carriage and waited until the boat disappeared from sight.

On the way across the Bay of Naples, the boy slipped into unconsciousness. His face grew pale and his lips blue. My grandfather could not have known that his son had a fatal influenza pneumonia. He did not despair, in spite of the boy's seemingly hopeless state. Communications were poor then and the war had made them worse. The four-and-a-half-hour trip on the boat had cut my grandfather off from news of the outside world. So it was with an enormous shock that he saw the streets of Naples jammed with people celebrating. An armistice had been signed. The war was over.

There he stood on the pier, with his dying son in his arms, facing a city gone wild with celebration. There were no taxis to be had, and even if he had found one, it never could have gotten through the crush. He set off on foot, making his way to the hospital. A few blocks from the center of the city, he found a horse and carriage and persuaded the driver to take him to the hospital. Some time during the next half hour his son died, just before they arrived at the hospital.

When the boat returned to Ischia on November 12, my grandmother saw her husband disembark alone. She knew what had happened.

On November 15 my grandfather began to feel unwell. He had a fever, sore throat, body aches and pains and a headache, all the unmistakable symptoms of the Spanish influenza. He was forty-six years old and strong and healthy. On November 18 he seemed to improve a little, but the next day he developed a high fever and had trouble breathing. He lapsed in and out of delirium, and his lips turned blue. On November 20 he died.

There were long-established customs governing funerals and mourning in Ischia. There were black-edged obituary notices posted on the walls, a funeral procession, tolling bells and floral wreaths. All of this had now been forbidden by the supposedly liberal government of Premier Vittorio Emmanuele Orlando in an attempt to hide the terrible reality of the Spanish influenza. So my grandfather was buried quietly and without display. Across the Atlantic in America, my mother and her aunt watched the epidemic rage from the seclusion of their home in Canton, Ohio. The schools had been closed, and people on the streets wore face masks. On the morning of November 21 a telegram arrived, announcing my grandfather's death. In Ischia, all of my grandmother's children came down with the flu, and before the month was out two more had died. Half a century later she recalled it all vividly. "That was the most horrible month of my life," she murmured to me "—my husband and three of my children."

Millions echoed her words as 1918 drew to a close. The pandemic eventually subsided and then stopped completely almost three months after it had begun, vanishing as inexplicably as it had broken out. The greatest medical catastrophe of all time had come and gone shrouded in mystery, and nothing like it has returned since. Could it happen again? Many scientists say it could. That is why there is so much concern over the Swine flu.

When the Spanish influenza disappeared, people lived in dread that it might return some day. As the years went on influenza did return, but in milder form, like the disease man had known for centuries. Pandemics occurred in the late 1920s, 1930s and 1940s but were pallid compared to what had happened in 1918. Then in 1957, a new pandemic started in the Far East, probably in central China. By April it was in Hong Kong, and in May and June it caused an explosive epidemic in Japan. As scientists watched its progress they came to call it the Asian flu. Before the age of air travel, the flu moved along sea lanes, roads and railway lines: one could map its daily progress at so many miles per day. But jet air travel changed all that. The virus was rapidly carried out of Japan to South America, Europe, Africa and the United States. This widespread seeding caused numerous epidemics to break out simultaneously all over the world. By August it was all over Europe, and by the end of October it had spread across the United States from Boston to San Diego.

This flu pandemic frightened both scientists and laymen who remembered the 1918 holocaust. It was much more severe than the flu outbreaks which had occurred in the intervening forty years. But it did not follow the 1918 pattern and return in a second, devastating wave. It primarily affected elderly people and school-age children, and the mortality rate was not as severe as that of 1918.

In 1968 another pandemic began, probably originating again in China. It was first identified in Hong Kong and for this reason came to be called the Hong Kong flu. Like the one of 1957, it moved rapidly across the world and primarily affected school-age children. It, too, was mild compared to the Spanish influenza. In 1972 came the London flu, another relatively mild pandemic, followed by a new Hong Kong flu in 1973–1974.

It might seem that pandemics are occurring more frequently than they did in previous centuries and in the early part of the twentieth. But this is not the case. Now we are more aware of minor pandemics, because of the sophisticated surveillance techniques scientists use to monitor the flu. This pattern of periodic mild-to-moderately severe pandemics continues. In 1976, for example, the Swine flu appeared and sent shock waves of fear through those who knew what its appearance meant. More about this in a later chapter.

CHAPTER V

The Flu Viruses and
Flu Vaccine

The havoc wreaked by the Spanish influenza spawned a frantic search for its cause in almost every corner of the globe. As the pandemic raged, scientists carefully examined the lungs and other organs of flu victims, cultured their breath and saliva in laboratories, and conducted innumerable experiments to determine how the disease was transmitted, how it could be cured and how it could be prevented. What came out of this hectic research was a morass of conflicting information. It was the age when bacteriology was still in its infancy. Virology had yet to be born: in 1918 a microscope could not detect viruses, nor had the technology been developed to isolate and grow them in the laboratory. Scientists naturally fell to looking for bacteria in the organs and cultures they examined. And find them they did. From this they naturally concluded that bacteria were causing the flu.

Early on in the pandemic pathologists and bacteriologists began to isolate one bacterium more frequently than any other. It was Pfeiffer's bacillus, scientifically known as *Haemophilus influenzae*. Dr. Richard Pfeiffer, the renowned German bacteriologist after whom this microorganism was named, first discovered it in 1892, two years after the 1890 flu pandemic passed through Germany. At the time of the 1918 pandemic, many experts assumed that this microbe was the cause of the flu. It is an organism that lives off red blood cells, and is extremely delicate and difficult to isolate and culture. No one was surprised, therefore, when it proved difficult to isolate Pfeiffer's bacillus from many flu victims. Although there was no trace of the bacillus in the lungs of some 1918 flu patients, its presence *was* demonstrated in the lungs of many others. Considering the delicacy of the microorganism, this was enough evidence to continue to support the notion that it was the real cause of the flu. But in London, several eminent pathologists were baffled. If the bacillus was causing the flu, why was it frequently not to be found when they conducted autopsies?

Some accepted the current explanation, which was that the bacillus disintegrated at the patient's death and thus evaded detection. Others wondered if their own laboratory techniques were not faulty. After all, there were prestigious medical centers where the bacillus was being found at autopsy in almost every case, and in the sputum and breath of live patients as well. At Camp Devens, Massachusetts, the point from which the flu spread to many other U.S. Army bases, the medical staff consistently found Pfeiffer's bacillus in the noses and throats of sick soldiers and in the blood, lungs, heart and liver of those who died. Across the world at the Peking Union Medical College, then run by the Rockefeller Foundation, American and Chinese physicians confirmed the Camp Devens findings. Impressed by this apparent consistency, lesser men were intimidated into believing in what was not necessarily there. At some centers the Pfeiffer bacillus was found in 60 percent of the cases, and at others, never. The negative findings were bothersome, but they could not be dismissed, since they, too, came out of the laboratories of highly prestigious institutions. In Berlin, Kiel and Frankfurt, the bacillus was not to be found—a weighty verdict, since at that time Germany was still the medical center of the world. Doubts grew until, finally, a sufficient number of doubting Thomases in the scientific world began looking for something other than Pfeiffer's tiny and delicate bacillus.

One of the first to question the role of the Pfeiffer bacillus was Dr. Emile Roux, then director of the Pasteur Institute in Paris.

He—and others—theorized that the bacillus, like the other micro-organisms found in flu victims, was merely a fellow traveler and not the culprit. To many this seemed a plausible theory which fully explained the contradictory findings to date. But it also meant that one of the worst disasters known to man was being caused by a totally unknown agent.

In the summer of 1918, Dr. Roux instructed Dr. Charles Nicolle and Dr. Charles Lebailly of the Pasteur Institute's Tunis labora-tories to conduct a series of carefully designed experiments to un-cover the real cause of the flu.

Roux had entrusted this task to two of the best scientists in the West. Both Nicolle and Lebailly were already well known for their studies of other communicable diseases; in 1909, Nicolle had proved that lice transmit typhus. For the new assignment, the scientists decided to conduct three distinct but interrelated experi-ments. In the first of these, they took human sputum from an army recruit in his third day of a severe bout of Spanish influenza. Then they swabbed this sputum into the nostrils of monkeys and dropped portions of it into the animals' lower eyelids. It was already well known by then that monkeys were susceptible to the flu, so they served as a useful experimental tool for studying the disease. Within a few days both monkeys were down with high fevers and running eyes and noses. They refused to eat and spent most of the day sitting apathetically. The period between exposure to the spu-tum and the start of their illness, plus the symptoms and the course of the disease, confirmed for Nicolle and Lebailly that the agent of the flu was present in the sputum of people who had the disease. Both monkeys eventually recovered.

The scientists then decided to infect human volunteers with spu-tum from a feverish case of the flu. Certainly questionable by today's medical ethical standards, such experiments were not un-common at the time. In fact, similar experiments had been con-ducted on a rather wide scale in Boston. Nicolle and Lebailly obtained two volunteers from a nearby army base and swabbed their nostrils with the infected saliva. However, prior to swabbing the men's nostrils, they performed the third experiment: they passed the infected saliva through a filter which effectively removed all the bacteria. Thus, if the volunteers became ill with the flu, it meant that something other than bacteria was the cause of the disease. Within three days, both volunteers came down with the Spanish influenza, and both, fortunately, recovered.

Nicolle and Lebailly now knew what Roux had suspected all the time: Pfeiffer's bacillus was not the cause of the flu, and neither was any other bacterium, such as the streptococcus, the pneumococcus or the staphylococcus. Many of these bacteria normally live in the noses and throats of healthy people where they do no harm as long as people are well. But when the host person has been weakened by a disease like the flu, these resident bacteria can attack and cause severe pneumonia and other infections. Any or all of them had been found in the lungs and other organs of deceased flu victims, giving rise to the theory that they caused the disease. Now Nicolle and Lebailly had shown that, rather than being agents of the flu, these bacteria were its frequent companions, causing what are now called "secondary infections" and showing up at autopsies. Whatever actually caused the flu had successfully passed through bacteriologic filters; this meant that it was extremely small, so small, in fact, that Nicolle and Lebailly knew they could never find it under their microscopes. On October 15, 1918, they rendered their report to Roux, frustrated by the knowledge that whatever caused the flu had come into their grasp and yet eluded them. Their findings were not accepted at all, but time would prove them right. The foundations had been laid for a great discovery.

At the time that Nicolle and Lebailly were conducting their experiments in Tunis, an agricultural inspector was making an important observation at the National Swine Breeders' show in Cedar Rapids, Iowa. J. S. Koen worked for the Bureau of Animal Industry as an inspector for its hog cholera control program. At this swine breeders' show, almost all of the hogs became sick, forcing the show to close prematurely. The swine lay in their pens, coughing and breathing only with great effort. Koen was an expert on hogs and their ailments, but he had never seen a disease like this in hogs before. Within weeks, it spread through hog populations all over Iowa and the Midwest. It occurred to Koen that this disease closely resembled the Spanish influenza then raging through many parts of the United States. He reported his observations to his superiors in Washington, D.C. and called the disease "hog flu." Many veterinarians agreed with him that the disease was new and unprecedented. But although they admitted that it resembled human flu, especially the Spanish influenza, they refused to go so far as to say it *was* flu. But Koen himself went several steps further. He posed a question to the experts: Are hogs giving the Spanish influenza to people or are people giving it to hogs? Koen's observation and question were as important as the carefully-conducted experiments of Nicolle and Lebailly. These two happenings were separated by both geographic distance and degree of sophistication, yet they were both crucial pieces of the great influenza mystery. Eventually scientists would tie them together. Years later, Koen's question would be answered. But in 1918, he was viewed merely as a pig inspector with a fertile imagination.

By the late 1920s, a decade after the experiments in Tunis and Koen's observations in Iowa, virology developed to a point where the technology existed for the discovery of the influenza virus. Dr. Richard E. Shope, an animal pathologist with the Rockefeller Institute, had taken Koen's theory seriously, and in 1928 began an intensive study of the Swine flu. He showed that the Swine flu was caused by a virus which often worked together with a bacterium known as *Haemophilus influenzae suis,* a hog variant of the Pfeiffer's bacillus. He found that the bacterium was not the cause of the flu in swine, but that it increased the severity of the infection. Thus, he reasoned that severe cases of the Spanish influenza were often those in which the bacillus was present. For unknown reasons it acted in concert with the virus to produce a severe, and often fatal, pneumonia. This mechanism by which two microorganisms work in concert, producing an effect greater than the effect either might have produced alone, is called "synergism."

Scientists today generally hold the Swine flu virus to be a direct descendant of the flu virus which caused the pandemic of 1918. For reasons which are not fully understood, it lost its ability to infect man for some fifty years, and until recently remained confined to pigs. Not everyone agrees that the Spanish influenza virus was the granddaddy of the Swine flu virus, but the direct and indirect evidence pointing to the connection is fairly strong.

As is so often the case in medical discovery, Dr. Shope's work paved the way for the eventual isolation and identification of the influenza virus. Using techniques developed by him in the course of his studies, three British scientists were able to isolate the influenza virus for the first time.

In December 1932, an epidemic of influenza broke out in England and Wales. The National Institute For Medical Research decided to attempt to identify the agent responsible for the flu; by this time virtually everyone agreed that it was probably a virus. The three British scientists who undertook the task were Sir Wilson Smith, Sir Patrick Laidlaw and Sir Christopher Andrewes. As the epidemic drew to a close in London, they took material from the throats of influenza patients and passed it through filtering membranes which allowed the virus to pass through, but held the bacteria back. They next infected all animal species that could conveniently be used in laboratory studies, including rabbits, mice, guinea pigs and rats. They also infected ferrets, because these animals were known to be very susceptible to the distemper virus of dogs, which causes a disease closely resembling influenza. The rabbits, mice, rats and guinea pigs showed no signs of infection and remained well. That meant that these animals were not susceptible to the flu and would not be useful in the experiments. The ferrets, however, had been inoculated in the nose like the other animals and within two days they showed unmistakable signs of influenza. But the ferret, though susceptible, was not a very convenient laboratory animal to use. So Smith, Laidlaw and

Andrewes went back to mice, and developed a method whereby they were able to infect mice and cause a severe influenza pneumonia in them. They showed that once infected animals recovered, they were immune to reinfection, and that the blood serum of recovered animals possessed antibodies against the virus. They also showed that the Swine flu virus and the one responsible for the 1932–1933 epidemic were related. The virus isolated by the British scientists was named "W.S." after Wilson Smith, the head of the team. In 1934, Dr. Thomas Francis, Jr., then with the laboratories of the international health division of the Rockefeller Foundation, confirmed the work of the British team and isolated an influenza virus from patients ill with the disease in Puerto Rico. This virus was called "P.R. 8." Influenza virology was still in its infancy and no standards had been established yet for naming influenza viruses.

Then came a tremendous breakthrough in influenza research. In 1935 Sir Wilson Smith and Sir Macfarlane Burnet discovered that the influenza virus grew and multiplied on the chorioallantoic membranes of hens' eggs. Now it was possible to grow and reproduce the large quantities of the virus that researchers needed to experiment with. The next discovery came in 1940. Dr. Thomas Francis, Jr., and Dr. Thomas Magill discovered a new influenza virus strain different from W.S. and P.R. 8. They called it the "Lee" strain.

Eventually the viruses isolated by Smith, Laidlaw and Andrewes and Francis—that is, the W.S. and P.R. 8 strains—came to be called Influenza A. The Lee strain discovered by Francis and Magill became the prototype of Influenza B. During the twenty years following Dr. Shope's 1928 study of Swine flu, enormous strides were made in the study of influenza viruses. The electron microscope was invented, and it revealed the variety of shapes the viruses took. Their complex inner structures were studied. But in spite of all these advances, no one could say with absolute certainty what had caused the Spanish influenza pandemic. The existence of the causal virus had not been suspected in 1918. And even if it had, contemporary microscopes would not have been up to the task of examining it. The nagging fear that this unknown virus might return prompted some scientists to launch a search to see if any samples of the virus had survived. The only place it could have been preserved was the Arctic. The scientists knew they might not succeed in bringing back live samples that could be cultivated and reproduced in the laboratory, but at least there might be some dead samples to examine under the electron microscope.

In 1951, Dr. Albert McKee of the State University of Iowa set out for Alaska with a team of scientists. By carefully researching records, they learned that an Army transport had set out from Seattle for Nome in November 1918, when the Spanish influenza was raging in the northwestern United States. Many of the people on board the ship became ill with the flu enroute to Nome. When they disembarked there, those who were very ill were nursed by Eskimo women. The disease spread rapidly among the Eskimos in the area, and within a few days large numbers of them perished. They and the soldiers who had died after arrival were buried in the perma-frost level of the earth. One of those who had died was a man named George Prosser, and thus the project to exhume the bodies that had been buried in the perma-frost for thirty-three years was called Operation George. Initial exhumations produced bodies that were not preserved well enough. But finally, Dr. McKee and his team were able to exhume several well-preserved Eskimo bodies buried in the tundra at Golovin. They took samples of lung tissue and other specimens and sealed them in sterile transport jars. The specimens were then frozen and taken to several research centers including the U.S. Army Medical Service Graduate School, the University of Michigan, Harvard University and the State University of Iowa. Elaborate studies were conducted, using ferrets, as Wilson Smith and his team had done nineteen years before. These tests proved negative, so other techniques were tried. None of them came to anything. The virus of the Spanish influenza had not survived three decades in an icy grave.

Influenza Type C virus was discovered in 1950 by Drs. Thomas and Francis. Shortly thereafter, a possible fourth type, referred to as Type D, was isolated. Since then our knowledge of the influenza viruses has steadily increased. Scientists have learned about many, though not all, of the characteristics of these microbes. The viruses, and especially the Influenza A virus, have two characteristics which distinguish them from many other microorganisms. Influenza viruses exist and multiply primarily in human cells, although some scientists theorize that they can also live and multiply inside the cells of swine or other animals. Influenza viruses are what scientists call obligate parasites; that is, they are almost always obliged to live in human cells and cannot live outside of them. Other viruses have more leeway. The polio virus, for example, can survive rather well in sewage; between human epidemics, the yellow fever virus survives in monkeys; and some viruses, like the one which causes chickenpox, can be latent in humans. Influenza viruses are delicate by comparison and possess none of these survival tricks—at least as far as we know now.

To be an efficient parasite, the influenza virus must live in harmony with its principal host, man. It infects the cells of man's respiratory tract, thrives and multiplies there, and in most instances does not injure its host to the point where he dies. If the virus were to kill its host most of the time, it, too, would eventually die out. So the influenza virus usually affects its host in a rather mild way, and its progeny are passed on to a new host via a cough and a sneeze.

Though having mastered this technique for survival, the virus continually faces a formidable obstacle: as it passes through the human population, man's cells build up antibodies to it. These defensive substances can destroy the virus in a matter of hours. If an influenza virus stays around in a community long enough, most people will develop these antibodies, and eventually the virus, which cannot exist except in man's respiratory tract, will die out. We know from practical experience that the influenza virus manages to cope with this obstacle in an interesting way. The viruses present in the respiratory tract of a flu victim at any given time are not all identical in terms of their genetic makeup. A single infection is caused by billions of virus particles. Some of these differ significantly from their fellows and are called mutants. These mutants are always around, but they cannot be detected because they are a minority in the influenza virus population. However, as antibodies build up and begin to destroy the dominant virus, mutants take over. These mutants are not totally immune to the antibodies that are destroying the dominant virus, but they can at least survive the attack. This phenomenon of survival is called "antigenic drift."

How is the ordinary person affected by antigenic drift? When drift occurs, the new mutant takes over the scene, and an individual who was immune to the old strain contracts the flu again. But since the mutants possess some similarity to their previously dominant relatives, they are affected somewhat by man's antibodies, and the flu they cause is often not very severe. Mutants tend to emerge every two or three years, and sometimes even within the same year.

Every decade or so, influenza pandemics occur. The viruses that cause these are not affected at all by any antibodies in the human population. This means that they probably did not develop in humans. If they didn't, then where did they come from? To understand the appearance of these new viruses you must first know something of the structure of the influenza virus.

Most commonly, the influenza virus is shaped like a sphere, measuring about .0000004 inches in diameter. Packaged inside the center of the sphere is the virus's genetic material called Ribonucleic Acid (RNA). The RNA is covered by a layer of protein, and this, in turn, is protected by a fatty membrane that has spikes projecting from it. The virus uses these spikes to get itself in and out of human cells. Once the virus gets into the human cell, its protein covering breaks down and its RNA takes over the cell and, in a sense, orders it to make new influenza viruses. When one influenza virus enters a human cell, it multiplies and thousands of virus particles emerge.

Many scientists now believe that the influenza virus may infect animals, such as swine. Eventually antibody levels in the human population become so high that a certain virus can no longer infect man, and is replaced by a mutant, as already explained. But it continues to be transmitted among swine and perhaps other animals, where it eventually undergoes genetic change. In time, the mutant that has taken its place in humans will infect swine and also be driven out of the human population by antibody levels. Inside the animals' cells, the mutant and its predecessor will combine their genetic material—the RNA—and the end result is a brand new virus, different from its two parents and capable of infecting man. This is the theory of "hybridization." The virus is said to "shift," meaning that it undergoes considerable change. This theory has been proposed by some to explain the appearance of pandemic forms of the flu every decade or so. They point out that the chances of this occurring are greatest in areas where there is close contact between man and domestic animals such as swine. Such close contact occurs especially in parts of Asia and it is of particular interest that most great pandemics have originated in Asia, probably in China, where contacts between man and swine are frequent and close.

As one can imagine, there is a very large number of influenza viruses, and it became clear to scientists early on that a logical naming system had to be established to keep them straight. This was especially true for the Influenza A virus which changes frequently, thereby causing epidemics and pandemics. The standards for this nomenclature system were finally agreed upon in 1949. Today each influenza virus is identified by (1) the type and family of the virus, (2) the place where it was isolated and its identifying number, (3) the year of isolation and (4) the surface antigens on the virus. Under the nomenclature system the Influenza A virus isolated in Victoria, Australia in 1975 is described as: A_2/Victoria/3/75 (H3N2). A is the type, 2 the family or subtype, 3 the identifying number, and 75 the year; H3N2 identifies the surface antigens of the virus. The major types of influenza viruses—that is, A, B and C—are identified in the laboratory by a test called the complement-fixation test. The families or subtypes, as they are called, are identified by the hemagglutination-inhibition and neutralization tests. To date, over a thousand different strains of the Influenza A virus have been identified. From 1933 to 1946 the first isolated Influenza A viruses continued to remain in circulation. They were called A_0, the o referring to the family of the virus. A_0 was replaced by A_1 strains from 1947 to 1956 and A_1 strains by A_2 strains from 1957 to the present.

In order to keep up with the new strains that are always appearing and must be identified, the World Health Organization has designated eighty-five influenza reference laboratories in fifty-five countries. Their efforts are coordinated through the World Influenza Centre headquartered in London. Each year the center screens hundreds of specimens flown in from flu outbreaks all over the world, to determine whether they contain known strains or new mutant strains. Similar screening is done at the eighty-five reference laboratories. Why bother to do this screening? It is done for a very practical and important reason, and it saves many lives each year. If a new mutant strain appears and causes an outbreak or an epidemic, it is important to identify it so that a new vaccine can be made at once. Vaccines that are effective against preceding virus strains do offer some protection against a new mutant, but often not enough—hence the constant lookout for new strains.

The search for an effective flu vaccine is a great saga of medical discovery spanning many years and involving several prominent scientists. Smith and Burnet began the story in 1935 when they discovered that the influenza virus could be grown in fertilized hens' eggs. Without this knowledge, scientists could not have produced a vaccine. Dr. Thomas Francis and Dr. Thomas Magill, who discovered the Influenza B virus, had observed that mice could be made immune to infection with an influenza virus if they were previously exposed to injections of the same virus. This observation, coupled with the discovery of Smith and Burnet, opened the way for the development of the first vaccines.

In 1936, a number of scientists began work on a vaccine. Some of the vaccines contained live flu virus; the rest contained virus that had been killed with formalin. When tested, all of these vaccines demonstrated two facts. Antibodies to the virus did appear in people who had been vaccinated—but not enough antibodies to protect them from a bout of the flu. By the end of the 1930s most scientists concluded that these vaccines were not practical preventives.

Dr. Thomas Francis had shown that antibodies rose to an effective level if a high concentration of virus was used in the vaccine. But unfortunately, such highly concentrated vaccines caused serious side effects. From the perspective of the person receiving the vaccine, it was better to get the flu than to get vaccinated. In 1941, Dr. George K. Hirst, now the director of the Public Health Research Institute of New York and chief of its department of virology, observed that the flu virus grown in fertilized hens' eggs could be separated from the egg product. Using this finding, Dr. Francis and Dr. Jonas Salk were able to produce the first concentrated and purified flu vaccine in 1942. The virus in this vaccine was ten times more concentrated than in previous vaccines, and consisted of the two strains of Influenza A virus and the one strain of Influenza B virus then current. Laboratory animals were tested, then large field trials were conducted among military personnel. These showed that the vaccine gave good protection for about a year.

Then in 1947, people who had been recently vaccinated began getting the flu. The Influenza A virus had shifted. A_1 had replaced A_o, and the vaccine made out of A_o virus gave no protection. This pointed out the necessity of constantly monitoring the influenza viruses. If a significant drift occurred or a shift took place, current vaccines became ineffective.

During the early years of vaccine development, the United States Armed Forces Influenza Commission sponsored and funded many research studies. From 1947 to 1957, these studies revealed no dramatic changes in the Influenza A virus. But then the Asian flu appeared, caused by a new strain, the A_2 virus. Vaccines then available gave no protection against it. Scientists came to realize that new types emerged every decade or so and that new variants of these types appeared every couple of years. For vaccines to be effective, the scientists had to be one step ahead of these changes, no easy task with only a murky crystal ball at hand. But through the eighty-five laboratories that work with the World Health Organization, new variants of the virus can now be regularly identified. The labs send any new isolated virus to one of the international centers to ascertain whether the current vaccines are effective against it. During the 1974–1975 flu season, the vaccine most widely used was a bivalent one, containing both A and B viruses. The A virus used in making the vaccine was the A/Port Chalmers/1/73 (H3N2), and the B virus B/Hong Kong/5/72. Those were the strains then current throughout the United States.

Only about three doses of vaccine can usually be made from one fertile hen's egg, so large numbers of fertile eggs are needed. The virus is kept alive in the laboratory, then inoculated into the eggs and allowed to multiply. Then the virus is killed with formaldehyde, concentrated and purified to remove as much of the egg protein as possible. The concentrations of dead virus in the vaccine are expressed in chicken cell agglutinating units, called CCA for short. Thus, in the 1974–1975 bivalent vaccines there were 700 CCA units of Type A and 500 CCA units of Type B.

Once prepared, the vaccine is packaged in bottles, usually containing 5 milliliters or 30 milliliters. The vaccine must be kept refrigerated between 35° and 46° Fahrenheit. Its temperature must not drop below 32° F., because freezing destroys its potency. The vaccine is injected either directly under the skin—a subcutaneous injection—or into the muscle—an intramuscular injection. There is evidence that side reactions are fewer when the vaccine is injected into the muscle.

During the 1950s, a person being immunized for the first time had to get two shots, two months apart. In recent years, the vaccines produced have been of higher potency, so one shot is now sufficient per year. The vaccines used today are usually bivalent, containing Types A and B. However, monovalent vaccines, containing either Type A only or Type B only, are sometimes made if warranted.

When you are vaccinated, you are standing at the end of a long chain of events. As you now know, laboratories all over the world identify new viruses and test vaccines against them. Pharmaceutical companies then begin to mass-produce new vaccines, using new viruses as they appear and cause widespread disease. But none of this can occur if flu cases and outbreaks are not monitored and evaluated. Flu surveillance is the beginning of the chain, and its methods are sophisticated. Scattered reports from physicians and the familiar comment, "Oh, there's a lot of flu around" can be helpful but are often inaccurate and impressionistic. Epidemic specialists monitoring the flu need much better information if they are to cope with a microbe renowned for its changeability and adaptability. A smart microbe cannot be outfoxed except by shrewd, efficient and precise detective work. To start the chain of events leading to the vaccination of your children and mine requires a detective system that tells disease specialists what the flu is doing every day in the general human population. Keeping track of the flu is a complex and difficult game, but one which has so far resulted in the saving of thousands and perhaps millions of lives.

CHAPTER VI

Keeping Track of the Flu

Each year programs are launched all over the country to vaccinate people against the flu. The stakes are large. Without vaccinations many people can become severely ill, and many can die.

For maximum protection, people must be vaccinated *before* the flu season, which usually runs from November through February and peaks in late December and early January. Vaccination campaigns are usually conducted in September and October. All across the country, from Oregon to Florida, mobile teams of vaccinators go into nursing homes and senior citizen centers. Vaccinations are given by private physicians in clinics, hospitals and health centers, so that the elderly and the chronically ill can be protected from the onslaught of the flu virus.

But no matter how effectively they are distributed, flu vaccines will not be effective unless they are kept up to date. The flu virus constantly changes to ensure its survival and the new virus strains have to be incorporated into the vaccines. So scientists must keep track of the flu. If they do not, the new virus strains can cause widespread and serious epidemics across the country, even among those who may have already been vaccinated against a previous strain. The costs in human misery can be almost incalculable.

Flu watchers keep track of three things: the progress of current virus strains; the size, severity and location of the outbreaks they cause; and changes in the virus strains. Such changes are suspected whenever there is a sudden increase in the number of flu cases and the number of related deaths. If a new strain is suspected, it must then be confirmed and identified so that new vaccines can promptly be made. The ultimate goal of all this medical detective work is to protect people from the flu.

Although individual cases of the flu are officially reported in some states, they are not reported on a national basis to the Center for Disease Control of the United States Public Health Service in Atlanta, Georgia. The reason for this is that so many other virus diseases mimic the flu. To be certain of the diagnosis, confirmatory laboratory tests must be conducted on throat cultures, sputum samples or other specimens. In most cases they are not; the local doctor makes his diagnosis simply on the basis of the patient's symptoms. Although the margin of error in clinical diagnosis is not great, most experts feel it is large enough to reduce the value of national reporting of cases. Therefore, other means of rapid detection have to be used.

For a number of years, elaborate flu surveillance programs have been conducted by certain city and state health departments, such as those in California and New York City. The national Center for Disease Control relies heavily upon the findings of these local programs. Prior to 1972, the Center for Disease Control kept track of the flu on the national level by telephoning state and city health officials to ascertain the level of flu activity during the fall and winter and by tabulating weekly the deaths due to pneumonia and influenza in 122 large cities throughout the United States. This system was too inadequate to last. The results of the telephone surveys were of uneven quality, since the various cities and states did not use a uniform set of techniques to gather their data. Nor could an up-to-date picture be based on the death figures from pneumonia and influenza. It takes about two weeks from the time someone gets the flu until he dies of the pneumonia complication, so these figures would reveal an upsurge or downswing of flu activity *after* it occurred. Scientists must have more immediate information if they are to move quickly against new virus strains.

In 1972, the Center for Disease Control began setting up a national program of influenza surveillance, incorporating activities that were already part of the surveillance systems in California and New York City. Forty-four states cooperated in the program at its inception and sixty laboratories forwarded the results of their analyses to the Influenza Center for the Americas, located at the Center for Disease Control. On the basis of their local findings, local public health officials were able to categorize the flu in epidemiologic terms as isolated cases, isolated outbreaks, regional outbreaks or widespread outbreaks. Any of the last three patterns were strong indications that a new strain had emerged.

The Influenza Surveillance System, as it is called, continues to operate intensively between the months of November and February, the so-called "flu season." Countrywide data is accumulated rapidly in a regular and uniform way and disseminated in *Morbidity and Mortality Weekly Report,* a medical publication sent out to all public health officials by the Center for Disease Control. The surveillance system works best in large urban areas of the United States. In some sections, such as in the north central and south central United States, the system works less well. The reasons for this have to do with the structure of the surveillance system, which I will now describe to you.

Whenever the flu enters a community, one of the first evidences of its presence is a sharp rise in the daily number of people going to outpatient clinics and emergency rooms of large hospitals. This is because many people in large American cities use emergency rooms instead of going to private physicians.

In other areas, however, such as in the north central and south central regions, it has been found that people are more likely to consult private physicians than to go to hospital emergency rooms or outpatient clinics. Thus the correlation between emergency room and clinic visits and the flu is not good in these areas.

In most states, however, several large hospitals are selected to provide the public health departments with daily and weekly rundowns of the numbers of people seen in their clinics and emergency rooms. This aspect of the system is called *hospital surveillance*. Through this method, changes can be detected in various parts of the country: a sudden and dramatic increase in the numbers of people visiting emergency rooms and outpatient clinics in a given city usually means that a flu epidemic is underway. The chances are that such an outbreak is due to a new virus strain. An intensive effort is made to isolate the new virus, and other states and cities are warned they too may be hit by it. Their own hospital and clinic facilities can then gear up to meet what will be increased demand on their services.

The second part of the national program deals with *industrial absenteeism*. Large corporations voluntarily provide state and city health officials with their weekly figures for the numbers of persons absent as well as the numbers of man-days of work missed. Whenever the flu hits a community, people miss work, so a significant increase in absenteeism is a strong indicator that a flu outbreak is occurring.

The third activity is surveying *school absenteeism*. Although the flu affects all age groups, the infection rate tends to be highest among primary and secondary school children. When the flu comes into an area, school and industrial absenteeism tend to go up simultaneously with an increase in visits to hospital emergency rooms and outpatient clinics. School absenteeism is a crucial indicator. However, in some large cities, particularly in the northeastern United States, the rate of truancy in the public school systems is so high that school absenteeism rates are of little help. Even in the absence of the flu or any epidemic, anywhere from 20 to 50 percent of the students may be truant on a given day. In some cities this problem has been overcome by surveying parochial school systems, where the usual daily absenteeism rate is about 5 percent.

The fourth part of the program handles *virus isolation*. During the entire year, nasal and pharyngeal secretions, as well as other materials, are submitted by private physicians and institutions to virology laboratories all over the United States. Flu viruses can be grown from such materials in either tissue culture or embryonated hens' eggs during the early febrile period of the disease. The virus can then be identified as to type, subtype and strain. The flu viruses are very elusive, and it is unusual that they are identified early on during an epidemic. Their identification constitutes a significant breakthrough, since it involves pinpointing the cause of well-documented epidemics. On the basis of that hard evidence, the pharmaceutical industry can then rapidly begin production of a new vaccine.

During the decade in which the Influenza Surveillance System has been operating in New York City, the flu virus has only been isolated once at the peak of an epidemic. This occurred in 1972, when the new London flu appeared in Europe.

On November 27, 1972, I received a telephone call at my office at the New York City Department of Health from Dr. William Braxton, the physician in charge of the Riker's Island Prison infirmary. He had called for some advice on how to manage a patient with viral hepatitis. The London flu was foremost in my thoughts, even though there were no signs yet that it was in New York City. Being a disease sleuth, I never passed up an opportunity to uncover the flu. So I said to Dr. Braxton, "Have you seen any flu-like illness among the prisoners?" He replied that he had noticed an increase in "colds" among the thirty-five hundred prisoners. "But," he hastened to add, "we see this sort of thing every year."

Although I couldn't be sure, I suspected that the increase in colds among the prisoners might mean that the London flu was in New York City. This was a new and fairly virulent strain of the Influenza A virus, first identified in London in early 1972.

"Do you mind if we come out to Riker's Island and examine the prisoners?" I asked. "Come on out," said Dr. Braxton. "But I think you're wasting your time. These prisoners have nothing but colds."

By noon, I was on my way to the prison, together with Dr.

Morris Chernack, who was chief of the Health Department's Bronx epidemiology division and Dr. Robert Harvey, who was an epidemic intelligence service officer from the Center for Disease Control serving in New York City. Once we got across the bridge to the island, it took us almost half an hour to get cleared by the guards at three inspection points. The infirmary building, a classic of governmental architecture of the 1930s, was dilapidated on the inside, with dimly-lit corridors, peeling green paint and stained tiled floors. We passed through two more check points and three sliding cage doors, and finally ascended to the third floor on a security elevator. After going through two more locked gates we entered the ward where Dr. Braxton was waiting for us.

There were fourteen prisoners in the ward, suffering from body aches, fever and headache. "I think it's the flu," said Dr. Chernack, as we examined the patients and their medical histories. Dr. Braxton disagreed. "I see this every year. Nothing more than a cold virus."

"Cold viruses don't put people into bed this way with a high fever," Dr. Harvey said.

In order to isolate the suspected flu virus we had to obtain specimens of the mucous from the noses and throats of the sick prisoners. This was done by having them gargle a solution and spit it out into sterile containers. The same solution was used to rinse their nasal passages. With specimens from ten patients in hand, we left the prison and drove to the Department of Health's Bureau of Laboratories on First Avenue. We handed the specimens over to Dr. Stephen Millian, the director of virology, for processing. "It will take about ten days for me to isolate anything," Steve said. "So be patient."

Dr. Chernack, Dr. Harvey and I had no doubts in our minds about what was out on Riker's Island. The prisoners in the blue uniform pajamas, tossing in bed with fever and body aches, could only have had one thing: the flu! But we had no proof and in our official report of November 30 to the Commissioner of Health were obliged to write under "Impression":

There has been no significant increase in the statistical data
to indicate the presence of a flu epidemic. The additional
absenteeism that might have been expected from the Thanks-
giving holiday did not materialize to any significant extent.
We are still awaiting the arrival of the London flu.

On December 8, Steve Millian, the director of virology, phoned
me, saying "It's influenza A," referring to the specimens from the
prisoners at Riker's Island. "But I can't tell you if it is the London
flu or not." To make a definitive identification, Steve had to send
the specimens to the reference laboratory at the Center for Disease
Control in Atlanta, Georgia. At the time, only they had the antisera required for identifying the London flu virus. They had not
yet made it available to local health department laboratories.

As things stood, we could not say that the London flu was in
New York City. But we strongly suspected it and knew that even
if the virus was not isolated from the Riker's Island prisoners, all
the flu surveillance indices—from the hospitals, schools, and large
corporations—would rise dramatically in a week or two.

At 3 P.M. that day, Dr. Rubin of the viral disease branch of
the Center for Disease Control in Atlanta called. "The viruses you
isolated are A/England/42/72," he said, giving the technical
name for the London flu virus. Out on Riker's Island, by this
time, four hundred prisoners were down with the illness; the
London flu had arrived in force.

The isolation of the London flu virus on December 13, 1972
was an unusual event in our flu surveillance program. In previous
years the viruses had eluded isolation and identification. The
presence of the flu in those years was deduced from steadily rising
statistics. But this year we had pinpointed the virus with accuracy.
Our discovery gave us a long head start on fighting the flu—and
doubtless prevented much sickness and death.

The fifth and last part of the flu detection system, and an important one, is *serologic surveillance*. When people contract the flu,
they form antibodies to the virus that caused their illness. These
antibodies circulate in their blood for years after they have re-

covered, and are capable of destroying the flu virus against which they were originally developed. These antibodies are also somewhat effective against virus strains that strongly resemble the one which caused the person's illness. However, they are ineffective against new and different virus strains.

People who are inoculated with flu vaccine also produce antibodies, and these are indistinguishable from those produced by natural infection. However, these antibodies only last for about nine months and then disappear. How does all of this help us keep track of the flu?

Throughout the year, blood specimens are submitted to public health laboratories for a variety of studies. On a routine monthly basis, samples of sera—blood serum—from these specimens are tested for the presence of antibodies to different strains of the flu virus. Such testing is intensified during the flu season. The results enable scientists to document which strain of the virus is causing illness and what proportion of the population is being affected by it. People who have received flu vaccine constitute a very small proportion of the population tested, so their high levels of antibodies—due to vaccine, not infection—do not interfere with the surveillance program. If a large proportion of a population is vaccinated, then serologic surveillance cannot be used as an indicator of what the natural virus is doing to the population.

One clear measure of the amount of influenza activity is an increase in the number of deaths from pneumonia. Pneumonia is often a complication of influenza; it usually causes death about two weeks after the onset of the original influenza illness. Death certificates are filed with state and city health departments and many departments tabulate the number of deaths due to pneumonia every week. The normal curve of this mortality statistic is a gradual rise starting in October and reaching a peak during the third week in January. Because pneumonia clinically causes death about two weeks after the patient comes down with the flu, an increase in the expected number of pneumonia deaths at a given point in time usually reflects the influenza situation of two weeks before. This information often comes too late to help in the fight against an epidemic, but the data is worth gathering, since it can confirm information obtained by the overall surveillance system.

The influenza surveillance system is the most effective means of determining the severity and longevity of an influenza outbreak. When absenteeism decreases and the pneumonia mortality returns to normal, it is evident that the population has formed antibodies to prevent further infection. The virus strain can no longer survive in the population. But when absenteeism and pneumonia deaths again increase, it is a sign that the virus has successfully evolved as a different strain or a mutation, for which present antibodies are not effective. Then the search for the new virus begins—the first step in developing a new vaccine. The influenza virus itself is elusive and difficult to find, but we can quickly learn of its presence across the country by watching for the shadow of illness and death that it casts.

CHAPTER VII

Swine Flu and
What Is Being Done about It

During the last two weeks of January 1976, Army medical officers at Fort Dix, New Jersey noticed an increase in respiratory diseases among military personnel. Some of those who were ill had symptoms compatible with the flu, and the Army doctors assumed that the Victoria strain of Influenza A virus, which was then causing outbreaks all over the country, was responsible.

The New Jersey State Health Department keeps the flu under regular surveillance and, as part of a collaborative effort with Fort Dix, took throat cultures from eleven of the sick soldiers. Seven of them, it turned out, had a Victoria-like strain of virus. Four, however, had a virus which was unlike those usually encountered in humans. It had the characteristics of the flu virus sometimes found in swine and other animals. Of the four soldiers who were ill with this Swine flu virus, one—an eighteen-year-old recruit—died of an acute viral pneumonia. None of the soldiers had had any contact with swine. This was unusual. It was not unknown for swine to pass their flu virus on to the humans who handled them. But the Swine flu had proved to be poorly adapted to man, and usually went no further than the swine handler. The outbreak in Fort Dix indicated a new and serious development—the Swine flu had become more adaptable, and was now passing from human to human.

In order to be absolutely sure that the Swine flu virus was the one responsible, the Health Department put the specimens through a battery of tests in two separate virology laboratories. They were examined under the electron microscope and tested against reference antisera. Reference antisera are obtained by infecting laboratory animals with a specific strain of flu virus. The animals then produce antibodies to that strain, and their blood serum—from which antisera is made—contains those antibodies. When an unknown virus comes in to an influenza referral lab, like the one at the Center for Disease Control in Atlanta, it is tested against antisera containing antibodies for various strains. For example, if the Hong Kong flu antisera kills the virus, then the virus has been identified. When the Fort Dix specimens were tested, the virus was eventually identified and given the scientific name, A/New Jersey/76 (Hsw N1). It is popularly known as Swine flu.

Once this virus was identified, a thorough investigation was launched at Fort Dix. This turned up one more confirmed case, bringing the total to twelve. Blood from 1,321 soldiers was then tested for the presence of antibodies to the Swine flu virus. Some 273 (21 percent) were positive, indicating that a fairly extensive outbreak had occurred. Many of the recruits who had the Swine flu may have had cases so mild they didn't even know they were sick.

The Center for Disease Control then launched a nationwide investigation to see if the Swine flu virus was causing illness anywhere else in the country. They found no evidence that it had occurred anywhere but at Fort Dix. An outbreak of Swine flu in humans had never been known to occur before. Fort Dix was the first case where Swine flu had ever spread from person to person.

The decision to immunize 215 million Americans was not arrived at lightly or without careful deliberation. On Saturday, March 14, a meeting of scientists from around the country was held at the Center for Disease Control in Atlanta, Georgia. Among those present were Dr. Harry M. Meyer, Jr., director of the Bureau of Biologics of the Food and Drug Administration, and Dr. John R.

Seal, director of the National Institute of Allergy and Infectious Diseases. They were informed that the Fort Dix virus had been found to be the Swine flu virus. For these knowledgeable scientists, the significance of this finding was apparent. It had long been accepted that the Swine flu virus is a descendant of the 1918 Spanish flu virus. Now it appeared that the Swine flu virus had passed over to man.

At the Saturday meeting a number of decisions were made. The initial findings that the Swine flu virus was the culprit at Fort Dix had to be confirmed in other laboratories; then a meeting of all manner of experts from all over the country would have to be held. Both steps were taken quickly. The findings were confirmed, and on Friday, March 20, 110 people met in Washington, D.C. to discuss the implications of those findings.

This was the first of many long meetings. Out of them came the decision to recommend mass immunization to the President. The decision was not clear-cut. At best, it was simply the safer of two choices. The Swine flu virus may never spread, but then again it may. Even if it does, it may be no more virulent than current flu viruses. The disease it caused among the Fort Dix recruits was not unusually severe. But as it moves through the population it could become more virulent, as did the Spanish flu, which was mild in its first wave and much deadlier in its second.

The full significance of the Fort Dix outbreak can only be appreciated by those who are extremely knowledgeable about flu viruses. Even before the Fort Dix episode, Dr. Edwin D. Kilbourne of the Mount Sinai Medical Center in New York City and one of the leading authorities on flu viruses in the world, had warned in a *New York Times* editorial that a new pandemic was on the horizon. In this editorial, which appeared on February 13, 1976, he warned that an imminent major mutation of the virus could be clearly predicted, and a pandemic would surely follow.

Is it all a gamble? Certainly—but in the view of respected scientists like Dr. Kilbourne, mass immunization is the best choice. Scientists will be accused of having cried wolf if no Swine flu epidemic materializes. If there is a flu epidemic due to a different virus, they will be accused of having provided protection against the wrong virus. And if a Swine flu epidemic does occur, some people are bound to get it anyway, even if vaccinated, since the vaccine protects 80 percent of its recipients at most.

In late March 1976, about a month after the Swine flu virus had been isolated from the soldiers at Fort Dix, President Ford held a news conference in Washington, D.C. He had met during the previous hour with twenty-seven health advisers, including Federal public health officials; well-known scientists; David Mathews, the Secretary of Health, Education and Welfare; and Dr. Theodore Cooper, the Assistant Secretary for Health.

"I am asking every man, woman and child in the country to get an inoculation this fall," the President said, and then revealed that he would ask the Congress to approve a $135 million bill to cover the costs of immunizing 215 million Americans against the Swine flu.

To go from an outbreak of twelve cases on a military reservation to the decision to immunize 215 million people is a quantum leap which puzzled many informed, intelligent people. "Is it necessary?" queried Representative Clarence D. Long of Maryland. A meeting of public health officers from states and communities throughout the United States was held in Atlanta at the Center for Disease Control on April 2, 1976 to explain the President's program. At this meeting, according to the *New York Times,* Dr. Martin Goldfield of the New Jersey State Health Department "questioned sharply the wisdom of pushing ahead with nationwide vaccination without any further evidence that the new virus is being seeded in the population."

Dr. Eugene Fowinkle, Commissioner of Health of Tennessee and president of the Association of State and Territorial Health Officers, supported the plan, but said that the amount of Federal money to be provided for organizing the program and administering the vaccine was too small.

"I question the national scare tactics that have been used," said a spokesman for the Wisconsin Medical Society. "I think they [the government] have overreacted to this thing."

"Our responsibility is prevention," said Dr. George E. Hardy of Birmingham, Alabama, president of the National Association of County Health Officers. He supported the program.

Skepticism was not limited to American physicians and officials. The *New York Times* had reported on March 26: "Officials at the World Health Organization headquarters reacted with surprise today to President Ford's announcement of a $135 million plan to vaccinate 200 million Americans against Swine flu virus. The organization said a month ago that there was no evidence that the virus which took 20 million lives around the world in 1918 was spreading. The officials declined further comment pending talks with United States experts on the project. . . ."

Less than two weeks later, however, the World Health Organization was taking a different position. The *New York Times* reported on April 9, 1976, "The World Health Organization said today that influenza experts had urged vaccine-producing countries to begin making vaccines to combat a possible outbreak of flu caused by the strain discovered at Fort Dix, N.J. . . . The twenty-two experts from sixteen countries who met here under the auspices of the United Nations health agency noted, however, that it was possible that the appearance of the new strain at Fort Dix was an 'isolated event.' . . ." The WHO said that in countries where supplies of special Swine flu vaccine might be limited, if available at all, contingency plans should be prepared to meet a "potentially exceptional situation." The experts urged "increased surveillance at national and international levels to detect any possible spread of the Fort Dix flu strain."

In early April 1976 Dr. Jonas Salk, who pioneered in influenza research before he gained renown for his work in developing a polio vaccine, came out in support of the President's plan. Earlier, on March 24, Dr. Albert Sabin, developer of the oral polio vaccine, had also approved the program.

But then, on April 6, the *New York Times* published a lengthy editorial in which it stated:

A systematic approach toward this issue must recognize that the President in effect made four assumptions in reaching his conclusion, and all are questionable. He assumed first that there is a real danger the nation will suffer a major epidemic later this year of a flu virus akin to that which caused the 1918–19 world pandemic. The President ignored the fact that most influenza deaths are due to bacterial pneumonia and other similar infections that can be combated by antibiotics, which are available now but were not available in 1918. The specter of mass death ahead is perhaps less fearsome than anticipated.

Second, the President assumes that the pharmaceutical industry can produce this vast amount of vaccine in a few months, and that all Americans can be vaccinated in a short time. Doubts are legitimate on both points.

Third, the President assumes that the benefit of a vaccine will be greater than its costs—in terms of human distress as well as money. Every medication known has unexpected side effects and can adversely affect those who are allergic to its constituents. It is conceivable that if there is no flu epidemic and if over 200 million Americans are vaccinated with this new pharmaceutical, a not inconsiderable number of people might suffer harmful effects for little or no gain.

Finally, the President is assuming that the vaccine produced will be effective, an assumption that must be regarded as questionable at this time when medical scientists have not yet even determined how much of the vaccine should be administered to each person.

The President's medical advisers seem to have panicked and to have talked him into a decision based on the worst assumptions about the still poorly known virus and the best assumptions about the vaccine, its timetable for manufacture, its potential for harm and its efficacy.

A convincing case for the President's proposal has not yet been made, and it cannot be made until those who support it debate publicly with the medical and scientific skeptics who are already voicing their doubts.

The call for public debate by the *Times* came too late, since the bill had already passed through the House Appropriations Committee on April 2. On April 13, the House passed the flu bill, authorizing the nationwide immunization program, as well as the other bill that appropriated $135 million to finance it. The Senate had already passed the bill on April 9, attaching to it a $1.8 billion Federal job program.

Why all this controversy? It all really started in 1918 when Dr. J. S. Koen sized up the sick pigs at the swine breeders' show at Cedar Rapids, Iowa and theorized that they had the Spanish influenza. Certainly, Koen never imagined that his theory would be proved correct by the learned world of scientists who have since studied the flu virus. And he could not have foreseen the day when a future President of the United States would call for the vaccination of every American against the descendants of the virus that had decimated the swine herds of the Midwest.

Dr. Richard Shope of the Rockefeller Institute spent more than a decade studying the Swine flu virus, and most flu experts then and now agree with his essential conclusion that today's Swine flu virus is probably a direct descendant of the virus that caused the terrible pandemic of 1918. Most of the great influenza pioneers endorsed this conclusion, including Dr. Thomas Francis, Jr., Sir Patrick Laidlaw and Sir Christopher Andrewes. Supporting their view is the fact that in the United States today, about 80 percent of the people over sixty years of age have antibodies in their blood to the current Swine flu virus. They probably developed these antibodies as a result of being exposed to the same virus in 1918.

Ever since the 1930s, then, when flu research was just beginning, most knowledgeable scientists have agreed that the Swine flu virus is directly descended from the Spanish influenza virus. But most of the general public, including many physicians, had never heard of the Swine flu virus until February 1976. It is worth noticing that support for the President's program came from the learned scientific community in the United States. Opposition in general came from those who are less knowledgeable about influenza. The President made his decision after being advised by a national committee of experts. It was their conclusion that the risk of an outbreak of Swine flu was real and that a major vaccination program was the only acceptable course. They conceded that it was entirely possible that no widespread epidemic of Swine flu would occur, and that, even if it did, it might be no different than the current flu.

Although they concede that an epidemic may not develop, the President's advisers do have strong evidence that it will. Swine flu has obviously adapted itself to the point where it can pass from one person to another. Also, it has emerged just at the time when a new, major pandemic-causing subtype of virus is due to appear. The Hong Kong flu subtype viruses have been around for almost a decade now. If history is as consistent as it has been for centuries, a new subtype is due to take over and cause a pandemic soon—and the Swine flu virus has already reared its head in New Jersey.

Some have said that the high mortality rate of the 1918 outbreak could not be repeated today. Millions died in 1918, so the argument goes, because they developed bacterial pneumonia. But today effective antibiotics are easily available—in the United States, that is—so even if the Swine flu did cause a pandemic, antibiotics could be used to ward off the complication of pneumonia. Experts are not soothed by this reasoning. If this is so, then why do so many people still die each year in this country from pneumonias complicating the flu, in spite of the use of antibiotics—one hundred thousand in the past eighteen years? There are two reasons for all these pneumonia deaths. First, antibiotics are not always successful in curing bacterial pneumonias. Second, some people develop a flu virus pneumonia that is not at all affected by antibiotics. Although it is often said that secondary bacterial pneumonias killed most people during the 1918 pandemic, there is no proof of this. That was the age of bacteriology and pathologists naturally looked for bacteria in the lungs of those who died from the Spanish influenza. They did not know of the existence of viruses, so they didn't look for them.

There are a variety of bacteria normally found in man's respiratory tract. Certainly some of them, such as Pfeiffer's bacillus, profited from the weakened state of flu victims and multiplied. But as pathologists of the day stated, the pneumonia of many flu victims was unlike any they had ever seen. It is probable that a good number of the 1918 flu victims died of a flu virus pneumonia and that the bacteria were mere fellow travelers. Antibiotics have no effect against the flu virus and would be of no help if a virulent pandemic broke out and caused flu virus pneumonia.

A whole other group of critics have challenged the feasibility of the immunization program. Can the country produce the materials and manpower this massive program will require?

The production of 215 million doses of flu vaccine requires from 50 to 100 million fertilized eggs. The poultry industry is able to produce that number. An industry spokesman is quoted as having said, colorfully, that it was rare that a program "both enriched the sex lives of roosters and helped prevent human disease at the same time." Four major American pharmaceutical houses are producing the new vaccine: Wyeth Laboratories; Merck, Sharpe and Dohme; Park-Davis; and Merrell National Laboratories. Two types of vaccine are being produced. One is a bivalent vaccine that contains the Swine flu virus and the Type A Victoria strain virus, which is the Type A virus still current in the United States. This bivalent vaccine is being offered to all those for whom flu vaccination is normally recommended, including all citizens over the age of sixty-five and people of any age who are suffering from chronic heart disease, lung disease, diabetes mellitus and other metabolic diseases. The other vaccine, which is being offered to the majority of the population, is a monovalent vaccine which contains only the Swine flu virus. As always in the United States, the virus in both vaccines is killed.

Many voiced concern that it would be impossible for the pharmaceutical houses to produce enough vaccine in time. But the pharmaceutical industry has said it can. On April 2, 1976 Mr. C. Joseph Stetler, president of the Pharmaceutical Manufacturers Association, told a Senate subcommittee that the industry would have 175 million doses ready by the end of the year. This would be short of the 215 million doses needed, but more than enough to immunize all who want a flu shot, since as much as 20 percent of the population may choose not to be vaccinated. They will still be protected because of the immunity built up in the country to the Swine flu virus through vaccination.

In an ordinary year drug manufacturers make about 20 million doses of flu vaccine. The drug companies have already produced 20 million doses of the A Victoria vaccine for the 1976–1977 season, so they are in a good position now to gear up and produce the Swine flu vaccine. Flu vaccine of the quantity needed has never been produced before in the U.S. But the drug firms say they can come up with the required doses if they keep their assembly lines running round the clock.

The safety of the Swine flu vaccine has also been questioned. Dr. Jonas Salk addressed this concern when he wrote in *The Los Angeles Times,* "We have been using flu vaccines for more than thirty years and side effects other than the occasional sore arm are very rare. The vaccine should not be given to people who develop asthma or hives when exposed to eggs; other than that I know of no serious contraindication. Infants and young children also require protection and can be given proportionally smaller doses."

The Bureau of Biologics of the Food and Drug Administration is responsible for licensing vaccines. Clinical trials in humans of the new Swine flu vaccine were undertaken in the spring, soon after the President's announcement. The bivalent vaccine, intended for the high-risk group, is being produced first, followed by a monovalent vaccine for the rest of the population.

One of the major criticisms of the flu immunization program is that it provides $107 million to produce the vaccine and only $28 million for the states and cities to do the actual vaccinating. At least twice to three times this amount will probably be required by state and city health departments. Vaccination via private physicians cannot be counted on too strongly. Vaccine is being provided to private physicians free of charge through their local health departments, and they are permitted to charge a fee for administering the vaccine, but not for the vaccine itself. However, it was learned in the early 1960s, during the polio campaigns when fifty million were inoculated, that public health departments had to vaccinate most people. As Dr. Albert Sabin said in Washington, D.C. on March 24, 1976, "Merely encouraging people to go to their doctors to get a shot would get a very limited response, as it has in the past." It is left up to the public health departments to corral as many people as they can—inoculating children in schools and dispensing free flu shots at special flu immunization centers set up in churches, firehouses, town halls and other local gathering places.

Health departments around the country have now geared up to meet the challenge, although many are unsure as to how successful they will be. The plan is that the entire vaccination program will be completed between July and November. Such a large number of immunizations cannot be given in such a short time without the use of automatic jet injectors. These "jet guns," as they are often called, can give about three hundred immunizations per hour without the use of a needle. The vaccine passes through a minute hole in the platinum head of the gun and is injected under the skin by the pressure of a hydraulic pump. During the spring of 1976 there were only 918 of these guns in the U.S. Two to three times this number are required to immunize 215 million people in four months. These are now being manufactured and should be ready by July.

A national influenza immunization program has been established within the United States Public Health Service, responsible for distributing vaccines to state and city health departments. Within the limits of the small budget provided by Congress, it is also providing some supplies and equipment and is giving small amounts of money for administrative costs. But the great burden of delivering this program has fallen to the states and the cities, many of which will have to curtail other services in order to take on this campaign. This huge undertaking is now underway.

Part Three

APPENDICES

The Anti-Flu Diet

Is there a certain diet that will fight off the flu? It depends on what you mean. There is no mystic combination of seaweed, organ meats, and Vitamin E that will flu-proof your body. But if you want to defend yourself against infectious diseases like the flu, start with good nutrition. The malnourished usually suffer more serious illness and run a higher risk of developing complications. In parts of Africa, the death rate for measles runs as high as 50 percent, whereas in North America and Europe it is a relatively benign disease. The difference is that in many developing countries the disease is superimposed upon already-malnourished children, whose condition is often apparent to the naked eye—swollen bellies, thinned reddish hair, edematous limbs and discolored skin.

Cases are not usually so severe in the developed world. But malnutrition is far from rare in the United States, and is not limited to poverty pockets and remote areas. During the past fifty years, the American diet has changed considerably, and primarily for the worse. We are eating more and more foods of animal origin, high in fat, like meat, eggs and whole milk products. People now consume more refined sugar products and eat fewer fruits, vegetables, and cereal foods. So-called junk foods are immensely popular, with all their saturated fat and simple sugars. Junk foods are "empty"—high in calories but low in vitamin and mineral content.

Yet they are sold in vending machines, restaurants, supermarkets and newsstands across the country. They are the most accessible and least nourishing of foods.

Running parallel to these developments has been a national trend toward physical inactivity. The less we exert ourselves, the fewer calories we need. But most of us are *not* cutting calories. As a population, we suffer from excessive weight, high blood cholesterol levels and a high incidence of coronary heart disease. Overweight people are not healthy people nor are they necessarily well-nourished people. They do not ward off infections as well as their properly-nourished counterparts.

A well-balanced diet equips the body to deal as effectively as it can with the flu. A diet of this kind was developed by the late Dr. Norman Jolliffe and his collaborators in 1957 at the New York City Department of Health. The Prudent Diet, as they called it, is intended for *healthy adults* who wish to have a well-balanced intake of basic nutrients—protein, carbohydrate, fat, minerals and vitamins. The Prudent Diet is *not* designed for people with medical problems such as diabetes mellitus and high blood pressure; they must follow special diets of their own.

The Prudent Diet will guide you to foods consistent with the American diet and steer you away from empty calories, saturated fat and cholesterol. It limits the total fat content of the food you consume and creates a more desirable ratio of polyunsaturated to saturated fats. The basic principles of the Prudent Diet are as follows:

1. Vegetables and fruits are high in minerals and vitamins, low in calories and fat and free of cholesterol. Include a lot of them.
2. Bread and unsweetened cereals are low in fat and are not "fattening" if you eat them in moderation.
3. Each meal should offer a protein of high quality. High quality animal proteins are fish, lean meat, poultry, low fat cheese and nonfat milk. Eggs are also high in quality protein, but you should eat no more than four a week.

4. Vegetable oils and margarines should be used in place of cooking fat.
5. Foods that are high in calories but low in food value should be limited. Foods high in these "empty" calories include candy, soft drinks, cakes, pies and pastries.
6. It is best to eat three meals a day. You can control your appetite better and utilize food more efficiently.
7. Adults should maintain a desirable weight. As we grow older, we should eat less, reducing caloric intake 5 percent for each decade between thirty-five and fifty-five and 8 percent for each decade between fifty-five and seventy-five.

To help you put these principles to work, below are listed the five groups into which all foods are divided on the basis of how much protein, carbohydrate and fat they contain. Also listed are the nutritive value of each group, and some general guidelines for its use.

I. Vegetables and Fruits

Cooked, raw, fresh, frozen or canned, vegetables and fruits supply vitamins and minerals. Green leafy and deep yellow vegetables furnish Vitamin A and iron, when they are not overcooked.

4–5 Servings Weekly, From These Vegetable Groups:
Dark green leafy: broccoli, kale, spinach, collard, mustard, turnip greens.
Deep yellow: carrots, pumpkin, sweet potatoes, winter squash

Daily At Least One of the Following Fruits:
High Vitamin C Fruits: grapefruit, oranges, tangerines, tomatoes, cantaloupes, strawberries, mangos, papayas

II. Enriched and Whole Grain Breads and Cereals

Although many breads on the market are almost empty of food value, enriched and whole grain breads supply B vitamins, iron and protein. So do cereals like oatmeal, bran and wheat germ.

RECOMMENDED	AVOID OR USE SELDOM
Daily servings of enriched or whole grain breads or cereals.	Baked products made with shortening or saturated fat: muffins, biscuits, Danish pastry, cookies, doughnuts, cakes and pies.

III. Milk and Milk Products

Although milk is no longer regarded as "the perfect food," it is indisputably the source of high quality protein, as well as calcium and riboflavin. Nonfat (skimmed) milk is best for adults; it contains all the nutrients in whole milk but little of the fat. Children can drink whole and nonfat milk. Some cheeses are much lower in fat and higher in protein than others. Check this list for the best choices.

RECOMMENDED	AVOID OR USE SELDOM
Daily, At Least One of the Following:	Whole milk (butterfat about 3%)
2 cups nonfat milk for adults	Cream, sweet or sour
2–4 cups whole and/or nonfat milk for children	Milk puddings
	Ice Cream
Buttermilk, low fat milk, evaporated skim milk (butterfat about 1%)	Butter
	Cream cheese
Nonfat dry milks with added Vitamins A & D	Cheese made from whole milk
	Non-dairy cream substitutes
Low fat, high protein cheeses: Cottage, pot, farmer, imitation process cheese spread (fat content not more than 5%)	High fat cheeses: cheddar, Swiss, dessert cheeses

IV. Fish, Meat, Poultry, Eggs

These foods supply quality protein, iron and B vitamins. Lean cuts of meat are best. If you are buying beef, ask for round, sirloin tip or rump cuts. For lamb, leg of lamb is best; for pork, loin, ham or leg. Chill soups and drippings to remove fat before using.

	RECOMMENDED	AVOID OR USE SELDOM
4–5 Servings Weekly:	Fish	Duck, goose
Often:	Chicken, turkey, lean veal (lower in fat than beef, pork, lamb).	Organ meats: kidney, brain, sweetbreads
4–5 Servings Weekly *:	Lean beef, lean lamb, lean pork.	Fat meats: bacon, sausage, corned beef, pastrami, salami, frankfurters, luncheon meats, spareribs, pigs' feet
Occasionally:	Liver Shellfish Dried beans and peas	

* One serving = ¼ lb. cooked meat
⅓ lb. raw or boneless meat
½ lb. raw meat with bones

V. Fats, Vegetable Oils and Selected Margarines

Some people mistakenly believe that they should eliminate fats entirely from their diets. Not so. Fats are essential for repairing and replacing cells and absorbing the fat-soluble vitamins (A, D, E, and K). Of course, only 2–3 tablespoons a day are required, but you should obtain this amount from polyunsaturated fats—which are supplied by this food group.

RECOMMENDED	AVOID OR USE SELDOM
Daily, From One of These Groups:	Coconut oil, olive oil
2–3 tablespoons (1–1½ oz.) of corn, safflower, soybean or cottonseed oil. (Peanut oil is not as polyunsaturated as these.)	Animal fats: lard, salt pork, fat back, butter, suet.
Selected margarines: those that list vegetable oil as first ingredient on label (ingredients are listed in order of quantity).	Vegetable shortenings
Products baked at home with vegetable oil, or margarine with a substantial amount of liquid vegetable oil.	Baked products made with saturated fat or shortening: cakes, pies, cookies.

The following guide can be used when planning meals.

BREAKFAST

High Vitamin C Fruit or Juice
High Quality Protein Food—cottage cheese, egg, fish, nonfat milk
Bread—whole grain or enriched, or cereal
Beverage

LUNCH

High Quality Protein Food—fish, cottage cheese, poultry, lean meat
Vegetables—cooked or raw
Bread—whole grain or enriched
Fruit
Beverage

SNACK FOODS

Various Highly Nutritive Foods
fruits and vegetables
nonfat milk
enriched or whole grain bread and cereals
nuts and peanut butter
cottage and pot cheese

DINNER

Fruit or Consommé
High Quality Protein Food—fish, cottage cheese, poultry, lean meat
Cooked Vegetables—high Vitamin A at least 4 to 5 times per week
Raw vegetable salad   Oil dressing
Potato or other starchy vegetable if you like
Bread—whole grain or enriched if you like
Dessert—if you like: fruit or fruit gelatin, pudding, cake or
cookies made with polyunsaturated oil
Beverage

SNACK FOODS

There is no guarantee that any diet will prevent the flu. But a well-balanced one such as the Prudent Diet will give you the necessary vitamins, minerals and nutrients that will give you better odds for resisting infection with the flu virus or for lessening its impact.

A Roundup of Anti-Flu Tips

Besides eating a prudent diet, you can take many other preventive actions during the flu season. Here are the ten most important:

1. Avoid crowds. Skip the movies unless you're dying to see the film. Walk to work, if you can, instead of taking a crowded bus.

2. Wash your hands often, especially when you return home from public places.

3. Move away from people who are sneezing or coughing, if you can—even if this means getting off an elevator or giving up a seat on the bus.

4. Avoid excessive smoking and alcoholic beverages during the flu season.

5. Don't get tired and run-down. Paint the living room *after* the flu season. Build a basement playroom in April instead of January. Don't clear out the attic or garage. For once you have a good excuse for not exerting yourself. Get plenty of rest.

6. Avoid close contact with anyone sick with the flu. Don't visit friends; call them up. Don't sleep with your sick husband or wife unless a hotel is the only alternative.

7. Obtain a flu inoculation *before* the flu season each year, if it is recommended for people your age or with your medical problems.

8. Keep children who are sick with the flu home from school until they have fully recovered.
9. Avoid prolonged exposure to wet and cold weather.
10. Use Vitamin C, if you and your doctor consider it effective.

Some Survival Tips
If You Get the Flu

1. Don't "wait and see." Call your doctor and follow his advice.
2. Stay in bed and get plenty of rest.
3. Keep yourself well hydrated with juices and soups.
4. Take aspirin every four hours unless you are allergic to it or it is wrong for you in some way. Also take Vitamin C.
5. Start on a bland diet as soon as your appetite returns.
6. Do not resume normal activities until your temperature is normal and you feel up to it.
7. If complications arise, follow your doctor's advice and take the medicines he prescribes.
8. Do not get up out of bed if you still have a fever, and do not go outside if your temperature is not normal.
9. Do not try to treat yourself with over-the-counter medicines. Call your doctor and get his advice.
10. Give yourself time to recuperate. Continue to avoid exertion, and get plenty of rest for as long as necessary. It may take several weeks.

ABOUT THE AUTHOR

DR. PASCAL JAMES IMPERATO is the First Deputy Commissioner of Health for New York City; he runs the Health Department. He studied medicine at the State University of New York and the Downstate Medical Center, and public health and tropical medicine at Tulane University. A diplomate of the American Board of Preventive Medicine and a Fellow of the American College of Physicians, he is on the faculty of both the Department of Medicine and the Department of Public Health at Cornell University Medical College, and is associated with the New York Hospital. He has written sixty-four articles for medical journals and is the author of a standard textbook on the treatment and control of infectious diseases in man. He has also written eighteen articles for nonmedical periodicals such as *Natural History, Sportsman, African Arts* and *Sign.*

Dr. Imperato is head of the New York City Swine Influenza Immunization Task Force.